EMERGING APPROACHES TO CHRONIC DISEASE MANAGEMENT IN PRIMARY HEALTH CARE

EMERGING APPROACHES TO CHRONIC DISEASE MANAGEMENT IN PRIMARY HEALTH CARE

Edited by
John Dorland and Mary Ann McColl

School of Policy Studies, Queen's University
McGill-Queen's University Press
Montreal & Kingston • London • Ithaca

Library and Archives Canada Cataloguing in Publication

National Chronic Disease Management in Primary Health Care Conference
(2006 : Toronto, Ont.)
    Emerging approaches to chronic disease management in primary health care / edited
by John Dorland and Mary Ann McColl.

Papers presented at the National Chronic Disease Management in Primary Health Care
    Conference, held Toronto, Ont., Apr. 6-7, 2006.
Includes bibliographical references.
ISBN 978-1-55339-131-9 (bound)
ISBN 978-1-55339-130-2 (pbk.)

    1. Chronic diseases—Canada—Congresses. 2. Chronic diseases—Treatment—
Canada—Congresses. 3. Primary health care—Canada—Congresses. I. Dorland, John,
1946- II. McColl, Mary Ann, 1956- III. Queen's University (Kingston, Ont.).
School of Policy Studies IV. Title.

RC108.N376 2006   616'.0440971   C2007-902425-4

CONTENTS

Synthesis and Conclusion

LIST OF TABLES AND FIGURES

TABLES

FIGURES

FOREWORD
CHRONIC DISEASE: OUR GROWING CHALLENGE

Michael Decter

In April 2006, I chaired a remarkable conference on Chronic Disease Management (CDM). Held in Toronto, it was sponsored by federal and provincial/territorial governments in Canada. Experts from across Canada and from the United Kingdom and the United States addressed the challenge of chronic diseases and their management. It was a very practical conference focused on successes, not theory. Even the tote bags handed out to conference participants proclaimed, "I made steps towards CDM Improvement." The meeting had that same practical direction to its discussions. While many presenters began with a theoretical framework, they quickly moved to sharing experiences. For an emerging issue such as the better management of chronic disease within health services, this practical sharing was immensely valuable. I am pleased to write an introduction to this book because it retains the same focus on how we can improve chronic disease management.

The reality of our time is that we are living longer, much longer, than previous generations. Yet, we are living longer not in perfect health, but with an array of chronic diseases such as diabetes, asthma, heart disease, arthritis, and others. Managing those diseases well is the major challenge facing aging Canadians. Helping us manage these chronic diseases is the major challenge facing the Canadian health system.

If we try to manage chronic disease in the existing acute care system, the most likely outcomes will be excessive costs and continuing health concerns. The struggle for both individuals and the system is to find better ways of managing these diseases. Fortunately, our motivation is strong as there is abundant evidence that better management equals better outcomes.

Prevention and healthy living are essential. The most evident finding is that active living and a nutritious diet help people stay healthy. Despite the best efforts of the existing health care system, millions of Canadians will spend one or more decades dealing with one or more chronic diseases. As Dr. Paul Wallace said during his presentation at the conference, you may spend 15 minutes four times a year with your doctor, a total of one hour. The other 8,759 hours a year you will be managing your disease! Self-management is at the core of the new and more successful approaches. Millions of Canadians will need to learn how to self-manage their chronic diseases. As patients, we are reluctant to ask our doctors how to cope with illness. We are much more comfortable being coached by a nurse or pharmacist. Apparently we are uncomfortable with taking the time of a busy physician. Finding a willing coach is one element of improved self-management. But as the conference indicated, a coach is not enough. There are specific and organized disease management programs that get better results than any other approach.

How much better are the outcomes from chronic disease management? By organizing more comprehensive care, it is possible to reduce hospital admissions, and significantly improve health outcomes with the support of a team approach. The really good news is that all across Canada there are innovative leaders in health care successfully taking up the chronic disease challenge. Moving these programs from the margins to the mainstream of our health care system is essential. Only a more robust and reordered primary care system of health care delivery can provide a proper home for well-organized programs of chronic disease management. The task at hand is to transform the overall delivery system based on the learning of early adopters about how we can do a better job.

If you have diabetes or asthma, or a family history of any chronic disease, you should be a strong supporter of these reforms. As individuals, we need to take responsibility for learning as much as we can about the disease or diseases that we ourselves will be managing for the rest of our lives. Understand that we will be the key managers, but that we can build a team to coach and support us. We must look for innovative approaches and family health teams that can support us to better care.

The conference filled me with respect for all those taking a leadership role in Canada and internationally to bring about needed change. It also filled me with optimism about the very real progress that is visible and the solid foundation that this progress to date has built for the future, larger scale effort. Only with a more robust and organized approach will all the benefits of modern health care be brought to bear on supporting those living with chronic disease.

MICHAEL DECTER is a former Ontario deputy minister of health, the author of several books on the Canadian health care system, and the founding chair of the Health Council of Canada.

ACKNOWLEDGEMENTS

The chapters in this book are based on presentations made at the National Chronic Disease Management Conference held in Toronto, Canada, on April 6–7, 2006. Thanks are due to many people and organizations for their contributions to the planning and implementation of the conference. Principal among them are:

- Health Canada, for essential funding through the Primary Health Care Transition Fund
- The Chronic Disease Management Steering Committee, and particularly Marsha Barnes of the Ontario Ministry of Health and Long-Term Care, for leadership and guidance
- The Canadian Federal/Provincial/Territorial Advisory Group, for supporting and facilitating Canada-wide project nominations and key stakeholder participation in the conference
- The Conference Planning Committee
- The many people who participated directly in the conference as Session Chairs, Moderators, and Recorders

Many of these individuals are identified specifically in the Appendix at the back of the book.

Additionally, the editors would like to express their thanks to Jackie Dickenson for her valuable assistance in organizing the materials and to Ellie Barton for her careful copy editing.

INTRODUCTION TO CHRONIC DISEASE MANAGEMENT IN CANADA

John Dorland and Mary Ann McColl

THE IMPORTANCE OF CHRONIC DISEASE MANAGEMENT

The management of chronic disease is destined to be one of the most significant health challenges of the 21st century. Driven by demographics and aided, ironically, by our past successes in treating acute health problems, the number of people with chronic conditions will continue to rise, as will the number of years that they can be expected to suffer from those conditions. Chronic illnesses often tend to be an unfortunate adjunct to living longer. Thus, in Canada and many other Western countries, increasing life expectancies combined with the imminent arrival of the baby boom cohort at the senior citizen threshold will generate an extra boost to the incidence of chronic conditions. However, chronic disease is by no means confined to the elderly. In the United States, the Center for Disease Control estimates that one third of the years of potential life lost before age 65 are attributable to chronic diseases. In Canada we see a similar picture: 57% of those under 65 live with at least one chronic condition.

While these conditions do not attract as much media or public policy attention as acute life-threatening illnesses, their negative social and economic impact is enormous. The World Health Organization (WHO), in a cross-country comparison of the impact of chronic disease, estimates that in 2005 chronic diseases accounted for 89% of all deaths in Canada. Furthermore, WHO predicted that by 2015, deaths from chronic diseases would increase by 15%, compared with a 6% increase in deaths from non-chronic causes. In economic terms, WHO estimated the loss of Canadian national income in 2005 from premature deaths due to heart disease, stroke, and diabetes at more than $500 million. In the decade from 2005 to 2015 this loss is predicted to accumulate to $10 billion. Although large enough, these figures nonetheless fail to include the undoubtedly significant economic losses and personal suffering from chronic illnesses in the time period preceding death, which by definition may be quite long.

Recently the needs of those with chronic disease have been receiving increasing recognition and attention from policy makers and health practitioners. Inherent in this attention is an appraisal of how well existing health care systems deal with chronic disease. In general, the conclusion has been that people with chronic conditions are poorly served by existing systems. The underlying cause is structural: a system designed to respond to acute illness, however well-funded, well-staffed, and efficient, cannot deliver adequate results in managing chronic disease. Even the basic language illustrates the mismatch: acute illnesses are *responded to*; chronic illnesses are *managed*. This recognition has led to the development and implementation of new structures and associated models of care, designed specifically for chronic diseases. These models are the subject of this book.

ORIGINS OF THE BOOK

The chapters in this book were originally presented as papers at the National Chronic Disease Management in Primary Health Care Conference held in Toronto, Ontario, Canada, on April 6–7, 2006 . The conference was organized by a national steering committee under the leadership of the Ontario Ministry of Health and Long-Term Care. Funding was provided by Health Canada's Primary Health Care Transition Fund (PHCTF) initiative.

The Government of Canada established the $800 million transition fund in 2000, in response to a national consensus among the provinces and territories that improvements to primary health care were crucial to the renewal of health services. Chronic disease management (CDM) in primary health care was identified by Health Canada and the Federal/Provincial/Territorial PHCTF Advisory Committee as one of the priority areas to be funded under this initiative. A wide range of projects were funded across the country to explore best practices and/or develop tools to support a collaborative team approach to CDM in primary health care. Part of the PHCTF funds were set aside to support change management by facilitating opportunities for sharing information and experiences as renewal efforts are being implemented. The conference received its funding from this source.

The conference brought together leaders in jurisdictions across the country to share experiences in implementing CDM strategies in primary health care. The main objectives were to

- explore effective practices that support a collaborative team approach,
- discuss common approaches and lessons learned from integrated CDM initiatives in primary health care,
- provide an opportunity for the provinces and territories to build a foundation for common approaches, and
- share the results of CDM initiatives across jurisdictions.

A steering committee provided strategic advice and guidance in planning and implementing the CDM conference. The committee was composed of experts from the field of primary health care and representatives from five organizations representing four jurisdictions:

- British Columbia—Ministry of Health Services,
- Ontario—Ministry of Health and Long-Term Care, Primary Health Care Team,
- Newfoundland and Labrador—Department of Health and Community Services, and
- Canada—Health Canada, and the Public Health Agency of Canada.

Selection of projects to be presented at the conference proceeded in two stages. Each jurisdiction in Canada (10 provinces, 3 territories, and the federal government) was invited to nominate up to five projects. Eleven federal/provincial/territorial jurisdictions (including Health Canada) submitted between one and seven CDM projects each for consideration. Based on a set of criteria coinciding with the conference objectives, a subset of the nominated projects were selected for possible presentation. A multidisciplinary committee reviewed the nominations using a two-level selection process. In the first level, the nominated projects were assessed based on the extent to which

- implementation occurred in a primary health care practice setting,
- interdisciplinary providers were involved,
- practice changes took place to better manage chronic disease management,
- lessons learned about implementing CDM initiatives would benefit other primary health care providers, and
- the project was systematically evaluated.

All projects were allocated an overall score, and projects with a score greater than 80% proceeded to the second-level criteria. Those projects that scored between 75% to 80% were reconsidered for inclusion. Among the projects scoring 80% and greater, second-stage criteria were applied to ensure that the final set of projects for the conference represented a mix of

- jurisdictions,
- chronic diseases,
- populations,
- geographic areas,
- best practice framework elements,
- stages of implementation and evaluation,
- organizations (academic, community based, etc.) involved in project implementation, and
- PHCTF/non-PHCTF-funded projects.

Out of this group, 20 projects were selected for participation in the National CDM Conference.

In addition to the Canadian projects, the conference included five keynote presenters. Three of these were international, from the United States and the United Kingdom. They were selected on the basis of exemplary success in implementing effective CDM programs in primary health care, in jurisdictions with relevance to the Canadian health care system. Two keynote speakers from Canada, from British Columbia and Ontario, were also chosen to reflect jurisdictions or models of care that were well established and had demonstrated preliminary results showing effectiveness.

In addition to the presenters, each federal/territorial/provincial jurisdiction was invited to nominate up to five conference attendees, representating relevant government decision makers, CDM stakeholder organizations, and CDM leaders and experts in the primary health care field. In total 110 participants from across Canada, representing all jurisdictions except Quebec, came together at the conference to share experiences, discuss lessons learned, and identify next steps in implementing successful CDM initiatives in primary health care.

THE BOOK

The book attempts to capture the breadth of CDM initiatives underway in Canada, as well as to showcase several exemplary international programs. It comprises chapters from all five of the keynote speakers, and from 12 of the Canadian CDM projects. However, as the selection process described above illustrates, these projects represent only a small minority of the CDM projects currently taking place across the country.

Michael Decter, the well-known Canadian analyst and writer on health systems, contributed the Foreword, based on his observations while chairing the conference. The succeeding chapters of the book are organized into four sections. The first is entitled "A Theoretical Framework" and contains only one chapter, a paper by Michael Hindmarsh describing the Chronic Care Model from the Group Health Center in Seattle, Washington. This model provides such a good overview of the chronic disease issue and has exerted such a significant influence over so many of the CDM projects that it deserves a section of its own.

The second section, "Leading Programs in Chronic Disease Management," contains four chapters on flagship programs that were featured in plenary sessions at the conference. They include two international papers, one from the Kaiser Foundation in the United States and one from England, plus two exemplary Canadian programs from British Columbia and Ontario.

The third section highlights "Canadian Initiatives in Chronic Disease Management." The chapters describe 12 Canadian CDM projects covering a range of approaches and chronic conditions. Each chapter is configured to describe the context within which the CDM program arose, the features of the program itself, the outcomes achieved, and the lessons learned.

The final section, "Synthesis and Conclusion," contains two chapters. The first, by Michael Hindmarsh and Nick Kates, summarizes recommendations that were generated in a concluding session at the conference. The second contains a summary, analysis, and concluding remarks by the editors.

Despite the magnitude of the problem of chronic disease as a public health issue, and the assessment that the current health system is poorly designed to deal with it, the tone of this book is far from pessimistic. Rather, the papers contained here are hopeful and inspiring. They document success stories and approaches that hold great promise for widespread improvements in dealing with chronic care. The potential benefits are huge; the required knowledge and techniques are available.

HOW TO USE THE BOOK

It is anticipated that there will be four main audiences for the book: primary health care providers, decision- and policy-makers, researchers, and educators. For primary health care providers, the benefits of the book are likely to be found in the various examples it provides of the application of the Chronic Care Model, and the experiences and problem-solving offered by these "early adopters." For decision-makers, the book provides a snapshot of the current state of the art in chronic disease management in Canada, and some basis for comparison of local initiatives against national and international developments. For researchers, the book provides some indications of the outcomes and methodologies used to evaluate existing CDM programs, as well as some benchmark results obtained. Finally, for educators of health care providers, the book provides a study tool to assist in introducing students in the health sciences to this influential new model of service delivery.

The book offers two additional features to assist readers in locating and understanding material that addresses their particular needs. The first is a set of Medical Subject Heading (MeSH) descriptors associated with each chapter. These are intended to guide readers to chapters that address their particular interests or needs.

The second is a brief glossary of clinical terms used in the chapters. Although this is not a clinical book, and the key themes relate to health system organization, delivery processes, and change management, descriptions of specific CDM initiatives frequently involve some clinical terms. Accordingly, we have provided a glossary to assist non-clinical readers.

A THEORETICAL
FRAMEWORK

1. THE CHRONIC CARE MODEL

Michael Hindmarsh

MESH HEADINGS
Chronic disease
Delivery of health care
Disease management
Models, organizational
United States

INTRODUCTION

In the United States, 63% percent of Medicare beneficiaries have two or more chronic conditions, and account for 95% of total Medicare expenditures. The situation is not dissimilar in Canada. As the population ages, we are seeing more and more chronic illness entering the health care system.

The increasing burden of chronic illness is evident in a 2001 (unpublished) survey of patients with diabetes conducted by Wasson in his medical practice at the University of Massachusetts at Dartmouth. Forty-five percent (45%) of the patients had additional diagnoses such as arthritis, obesity, hypertension, and cardiovascular disease; 50% had functional limitations that were emotional or physical, and that restricted activities of daily life; 35% presented with more than two symptoms, such as eating or weight problems, joint pain, sleep disorders or dizziness, and fatigue; and 30% had poor lifestyle habits, such as poor diet, poor exercise, or substance abuse problems.

For people over the age of 50, their most pressing concerns are about chronic illness, and their biggest fears are losing independence, being a burden to their family or friends, not receiving care in a timely fashion, and not being able to afford medications.

These data illustrate that as the population ages, our health care system is not able to handle this burden of chronic disease. The current system was designed in the mid-1900s to deal with infectious disease and injuries. Its focus is on managing short-term problems in the most expedient fashion, which has typically been the 15-minute face-to-face visit. As we push more and more people with chronic illness through this system, it cannot manage these patients effectively. The result is that outcomes for patients with chronic illness are very poor:

- Less than 10% of patients with diabetes receive the four basic guidelines of care—annual eye and foot exams, blood sugar testing at least once a year, and renal screening.
- Only 48% of patients with asthma are taking their medications properly.
- Only 60% of patients, 65 years or older, with a history of myocardial infarction are on statins.
- Only 25% of hypertensive patients have their disease under control.
- Less than 50% of patients with clinically significant depression are treated properly.

It is safe to say that the current health care system is perfectly designed to get these results and it can do no better. Asking providers to work harder or admonishing patients to be more compliant will not work. What is needed is fundamental system change to develop proactive care that meets the needs of chronically ill patients.

There are a number of problems with current disease management efforts. First, they focus on physician behaviour, not system change. Additionally, characteristics of successful interventions are not categorized usefully in the research literature, thus making it very difficult for care providers to know what is the best care to deliver. Finally, commonalities across chronic conditions have been unappreciated, resulting in disease-specific programs with differing infrastructures and modes of implementation that tax the primary care system. What is needed is a single system of care with a common infrastructure for all chronic care needs. That is the premise behind the Chronic Care Model (Figure 1.1).

THE CHRONIC CARE MODEL

The Chronic Care Model originated in the early 1990s with attempts to improve care for diabetes at the Group Health Cooperative (GHC) in Seattle, Washington, which has approximately 20,000 patients with diabetes. Similar improvement efforts were running concurrently for heart care, smoking cessation, prenatal care, depression, and asthma. Each effort came with its own infrastructure and separate program elements. It became clear that multiple disease-focused efforts were inefficient and impossible to implement at the primary care level.

To remedy this, our team at the MacColl Institute for Healthcare Innovation, a research arm of GHC, carefully reviewed the literature on chronic care and posited the first version the Chronic Care Model in 1995 under the leadership of the institute's director, Ed Wagner. In 1996, GHC was funded (by the Robert Wood Johnson Foundation) to bring together international experts in chronic illness care to further refine the model. The MacColl team convened the experts, elicited their suggestions for programs that they believed were already delivering model-based care, and visited the 72 suggested programs to test the model against these programs. We observed that programs

Figure 1.1
The Chronic Care Model

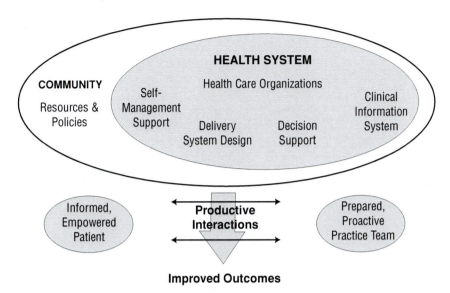

Note: Overview of the Chronic Care Model, from the Improving Chronic Illness Care website (n.d.). Retrieved March 4, 2007, from http://www.improvingchroniccare.org/change/model/ components.html. Copyright 1998 by ACP-ASIM Journals and Books. Reprinted with permission.

that had elements of care spanning the six major components of the model had better outcomes than those that had only some elements of the model.

PRODUCTIVE INTERACTIONS BETWEEN PATIENTS AND PROVIDERS

The six components of the model are discussed below, but first it is important to clarify the nature of a productive interaction between patients and providers. Current interactions tend to be frustrating for both parties. Patients find it difficult to access their providers and, when they do, feel the need to accomplish everything in one visit. When all their needs are not met, they leave the interaction unsatisfied. Providers typically do not have the time to deliver all the chronic care needs for the patient and will "symptom-swat" or address only the presenting complaint. They hurry through the visit, which often ends in doling out a prescription and pamphlets on improving lifestyle. Like the patient, the provider is unsatisfied with the nature of the interaction, wishes that more could have been done, and worries about what might not have been done.

   A productive interaction requires an informed, activated patient on one side and a prepared, proactive team on the other. The informed, activated patient is one who understands his or her disease process and is empowered as a self-manager of care. Such a patient takes advantage of the clinician's medical expertise rather than assuming the clinician will "fix" him or her. Family and caregivers are equally involved in the management of the patient's care.

A prepared, proactive practice team is one that has the right information, equipment, and personnel at the time of the visit. Appropriate decision support is easily accessible in order to deliver evidence-based clinical care and self-management support. The productive interaction is one where all clinical and behavioural assessments are available prior to the visit. The provider understands the patient's confidence level in managing his or her chronic condition. Clinical care is tailored by a stepped protocol. Collaborative goal setting and problem solving results in a shared care plan that both patient and provider understand. Critically, there is active, sustained follow-up to ensure the patient can manage the treatment plan and engage in improved self-management support.

REDESIGNING THE SYSTEM OF CARE

In order to get to this productive interaction, the health care system must redesign itself according to the six components of the Chronic Care Model (see Figure 1.1).

1. Health Care Organization

If chronic care is to be improved in any organization, there must be committed leadership that visibly supports quality improvement at all levels. Chronic care improvement should be part of the business plan, not just the quality plan. Performance incentives need to be available for care teams; they can be either financial or capacity building. Errors should be handled openly and systematically so that the organization can learn from its mistakes. Furthermore, care coordination agreements must be developed across settings to ensure smooth transitions for patients and providers.

2. Community Resources

The health care organization resides in a larger community with resources and policies that can support patients in meeting the goals of their care plans. Since the organization cannot be all things to all patients, it should refer patients to these resources to ensure they receive support to manage their illness. Examples include forming relationships with community or fitness centres to provide exercise support, or engaging public health organizations to provide nutritional information and diet coaching. Where such resources do not exist, the organization should form community partnerships to create programs.

3. Self-Management Support

Self-management support is the process by which patients learn to cope with the emotional and physical changes that come with their chronic condition.

The goal is for the patient to be able to carry out activities of normal daily life. It is not sufficient to simply educate patients about their chronic illness; they must be provided with the skills and tools to change lifestyle behaviours and improve outcomes. To this end, the care team is responsible for introducing the concept of self-management support to patients, and empowering them as self-managers. It is also the care team's responsibility to support patients' self-management at every visit. As Bodenheimer said at a presentation to members of the California Public Hospital Chronic Disease Collaborative in 2005, "self-management is inevitable." The task of the health care team is to help patients' self-management in the most beneficial manner.

4. Delivery System Design

To move beyond the current reactive, acute care model, providers will need to function in multidisciplinary care teams. The professionals on these teams can no longer operate in isolation, but must work together with clear roles and responsibilities for managing chronic illness care. Much like the well-defined protocols for a patient who presents with a laceration to the arm, the primary care team needs to be organized with defined roles and tasks for managing patients with chronic illness. Additionally, the team must set aside time to meet to discuss patient care. This can be done through short huddles at the beginning of the day and/or through weekly meetings where enough time is set out to discuss cases and plan for improvements in the practice.

With a team in place, care can now be delivered in a planned fashion. Planned care involves visits generated by the practice. These visits are designed to focus solely on the patient's chronic care issues. The team proactively reaches out to patients to bring them in for these visits, and expectations for visit structure and content are agreed upon between patient and the team. The team prepares for the visit by reviewing the medical record for needed care and ordering labs ahead of time. These visits can be done in the traditional one-on-one format or through group visits. The key concept is that the visit is anticipated and planned for. There is a clear process with well-defined roles and responsibilities, so that neither patient nor providers are surprised.

Another piece of delivery system design is the need for clinical case management. A certain percentage of patients who are at risk for complications will need more intensive management than the primary care team can deliver. Clinical case management ensures that the patient receives intensive support and follow-up. Most importantly, the case manager has direct access to the primary care team should there be changes to medication regimens or other aspects of the treatment plan. The case manager also helps the patient navigate through the health system to ensure smooth transitions between care settings.

Proactive and sustained follow-up that happens at regular intervals is another system change the care team must ensure. Without a system of follow-up, patients are likely to slip through the cracks or not contact the care team until they are in trouble. A care team member (perhaps an administrative staff member) needs dedicated time to do follow-up calls or emails to check on patients' progress.

The final delivery system change is the need to deliver care in a fashion that patients understand and that fits with their culture. This does not mean that care teams need to speak 140 different languages! It means that the care team must be sensitive to cultural differences and be prepared to discuss these differences with patients to foster comfort between both parties.

5. Decision Support

It is imperative that evidence-based guidelines be embedded in practice so that it is virtually impossible not to deliver the right care. Guidelines should be simple, easy to use, and readily available at the time of the visit. One way to reinforce guideline-based care is to change the relationship between specialty care and primary care. There is a need to move beyond the traditional referral model where patients go out to specialty care, and return some indefinite period of time later with little or no information transferred to the primary care provider about the improvements made in care. Care agreements between specialty and primary care providers that ensure a two-way flow of information are needed. That way the specialist knows exactly why the patient is being referred. Similarly, the specialist agrees to provide the necessary information to the primary care team so it can learn to manage care better in the future. If possible, the primary care provider and the specialist should jointly visit patients with complex conditions, so that the primary care provider can benefit from the specialist's expertise in a "hands-on" way.

To foster change in practice behaviour, continuing medical education, while necessary, is not sufficient. Provider teams need to engage in proven educational methods that are action oriented. They must be able to work with their own data and patient populations in order to move from the theoretical to the practical.

Finally, the care team needs to share guidelines with patients. If patients understand why a test or a procedure is being ordered and how it fits within their care plan, they are more likely to comply with the care team's recommendations.

6. Clinical Information Systems

Clinical information technology (IT) is the glue that holds practice redesign together. The practice team cannot improve care for its patients if it does not know who they are. The information system should not only support individual planned care, but must also be able to identify populations of patients for outreach. This kind of functionality is often referred to as a registry, and it allows the practice team to stratify populations according to risk levels and care needs. If the practice is using an electronic medical record, the system must carry this population-based functionality. The information system must also provide timely reminders to both providers and patients about needed care.

If possible, the system should be able to produce patient summaries for use at the time of the visit. These summaries can be used as care reminders and make the visit more efficient. In addition to showing outcome data to patients such as blood pressure or lipids, over time the use of summaries increases patient understanding of the disease process and helps the provider link patient self-management behaviour to outcomes. Clinical IT also provides performance measurement data so that the care team members can track their progress as they engage in quality improvement.

EVIDENCE SUPPORTING THE CHRONIC CARE MODEL

There are a number of advantages to using the Chronic Care Model as a system redesign strategy. Once the model is applied to a single condition, the infrastructure required at the practice level to manage any chronic condition is in place. All that is needed to tackle another condition are condition-specific guidelines, protocols, and self-management behaviours. The Chronic Care Model works equally well for preventive care as it does for chronic care, and it provides a mechanism for diagnosing the health system's proficiencies and inefficiencies so that quality improvement can be targeted where it is needed most. The Chronic Care Model has been applied to numerous conditions, including diabetes, congestive heart failure, asthma, depression, HIV, primary prevention, and geriatric care.

There are numerous studies of systems implementing the Chronic Care Model, few of which are randomized controlled trials. Studies representative of most of the literature on the effectiveness of the model have been conducted by the RAND Corporation, an American-based nonprofit research institution, and by the MacColl Institute.

In order to assess to what extent the Chronic Care Model improves outcomes, the RAND Corporation (n.d.) conducted an independent evaluation of U.S. chronic care collaboratives to determine whether participating organizations were able to successfully implement all components of the model and make significant, systemic changes that improved processes and clinical outcomes. The study was a pre/post-controlled design with 34 practice teams from various organizations in the intervention arm, and 24 controls from the same organizations. It involved medical record reviews, provider interviews, patient surveys, and automated data collection. The study examined three disease populations: diabetes, asthma, and congestive heart failure.

- For diabetes, while there were not significant differences in hemoglobin A1C, there were improved A1Cs in both interventions and controls, due in large part to contamination of the controls by their intervention counterparts at the clinic sites.
- For congestive heart failure, there were significant improvements in counselling and patient education, and reduced readmissions to emergency rooms.
- For asthma, there were significant improvements in the number of patients on controller medications and in quality of life.

The MacColl Institute has conducted numerous studies on learning collaboratives in recent years. The collaboratives involve 15 to 50 primary practice teams that meet for three two-day sessions over the course of a year. They learn about the Chronic Care Model and effective quality improvement strategies, and work collaboratively to develop improvement plans. Between sessions they test those ideas for change in their practice, and collect data to measure improvements. These data are shared with other participants in the later sessions. On average, 70% of teams created system change that improved both process and clinical outcomes:

• Twice as many patients with major depression recovered in 6 months.
• Inner city kids with moderate or severe asthma had 13 or fewer days per year with symptoms.
• Readmission rates of patients hospitalized with congestive heart failure were cut nearly in half.

One of the most notable set of learning collaboratives is the U.S. Bureau of Primary Healthcare's Health Disparities Collaboratives. The Bureau oversees the 850 federally funded community health clinics in the United States that serve the poor and uninsured. Results to date suggest that there have been significant improvements in processes of care for patients with diabetes, asthma, cardiovascular disease, depression, and HIV.

INTERNATIONAL PERSPECTIVES

The World Health Organization (WHO) has noted the increasing burden of chronic disease in developing countries. WHO has adopted the Chronic Care Model, adapting it significantly to fit the governmental and policy structures of most developing countries. The major focus is to create positive policy environments that promote consistent financing and develop the needed human resources to deliver chronic care. The WHO model also places greater emphasis on the community to raise awareness and reduce stigma of some chronic diseases. The model predicts better outcomes through effective leadership and support, and mobilizing/coordinating resources at the community level to ensure all services are provided.

The National Health System (NHS) in the United Kingdom (see chapter 5) draws upon the Chronic Care Model and the Kaiser pyramid. The key components of the NHS model focus on linking the health care system with the social care system. It places the patients and their caregivers at the centre of that relationship. The model is targeting long-term conditions, and risk-stratifying chronically ill patients for targeted interventions with an emphasis on frequent users. Multidisciplinary teams are being developed in primary care, supported by "matron" or nurse-led case management. There is local self-management support at the primary care level as well as the creation of community-based programs.

In Europe, a number of countries have also adopted components of the Chronic Care Model. Many of them had elements of model care in place prior to the development of the Chronic Care Model. For example, France has been voted the number one health care system by the WHO and has health care costs half that of the United States due in large part to their success at ensuring care coordination across settings. Denmark, Netherlands, Germany, and Italy have also implemented components of the model, specifically around self-management support, care coordination, group visits, and partnering with community resources.

New Zealand's Medical Outcomes Intervention is using the Chronic Care Model in an attempt to divert hospital use as the primary care medical home. It has also incorporated aspects of the Life Course Model, which acknowledges the social determinants of health. The determinants are used to tailor medical care and self-management.

Australia's Chronic Disease Model for Prevention and Control (again based on the Chronic Care Model) has been in place since 2001. It's a public health model that attempts to target and stratify chronically ill patients and match them to the appropriate services. Their approach is similar to that of the NHS in the United Kingdom.

CONCLUSION

The Chronic Care Model is proving to be an effective strategy for implementing comprehensive health system change. It addresses the dysfunction of the current acute care system, not by tweaking away at its deficiencies, but by establishing a new system of care that meets the unique needs of the chronically ill. While implementing the model is challenging work, thousands of health care organizations around the world are succeeding and demonstrating improved outcomes.

REFERENCES

Improving Chronic Illness Care. (n.d.). The Chronic Care Model. Retrieved March 4, 2007, from http://www.improvingchroniccare.org/change/model/components/html
RAND Corporation. (n.d.). Improving chronic illness care evaluation. Retrieved March 3, 2007, from http://www.rand.org/health/projects/icice/

LEADING PROGRAMS IN CHRONIC DISEASE MANAGEMENT

2. IMPROVING POPULATION HEALTH AND CHRONIC DISEASE MANAGEMENT

Paul Wallace and Joshua Seidman

MESH HEADINGS
Case management
Chronic disease
Disease management
Health promotion
Models, organizational
Risk
Risk factors
Self-care
United States

BACKGROUND

One of the greatest economic and quality-of-care challenges facing the health care system is how we manage chronic care for an aging population. The reality of limited resources and changing demographics means that simply stretching the "sick-care" system of physician visits further is unfeasible. With a population increasingly in need of chronic illness care, how does our society efficiently address these broad needs? The answer to this conundrum lies in shifting our view of health care. Instead of viewing acute care and public health activities as opposite ends of a spectrum, the new paradigm of health care places the locus of control with the individual, and care delivery migrates to prospectively meet individual needs. By bridging the gap between dealing with the individual's immediate symptoms and managing the population's long-term health, we restore balance to chronic care and promote improvements in both costs and outcomes.

Historically, the health care system has been designed primarily to deliver sick care on the one hand and to address public health on the other. While both avenues have yielded important successes, chronic disease management addresses the "middle space," bridging the continuum of care between the two traditional approaches and drawing on their complementary strengths: personalized access to optimal medical expertise, and the systemic capacity to meet broad population- and community-based needs. Many activities can thrive in this middle ground, and most of them rely on linking systems of care with individual needs over time. Bridging those concepts requires development of "mass-customized" interventions, or what others have called "mass personalization" (Christopherson, 2004). Success also involves leveraging a team concept for developing and delivering necessary care capacity and capabilities.

In seeking to improve the care for individuals with chronic conditions such as heart disease and diabetes, the initial attempts at chronic disease management have generally involved identifying the sickest people with a particular chronic disease and then taking an aggressive approach to case management. Over time, however, there has been an increased recognition that chronic patients often cannot be best classified as having a distinct disease, but rather as having multiple, often related, chronic conditions (e.g., the increasingly common individual who lives with both diabetes and coronary artery disease). In addition, it has become clear that solitary reliance on the hierarchal physician-patient relationship has not only stressed providers, but has also failed to tap one of the most influential components of chronic care management—active self-management by the patient. A growing body of research has demonstrated the degree to which consumers can and are using carefully targeted health information to manage their conditions. With the right support and infrastructure, such interventions have been shown to improve health, with the promise of long-term, efficient use of resources. Finally, appropriately prescribed and accessible information supports the active involvement of the patient and is an effective response to the growing recognition that a broad spectrum of care needs exists throughout any given population.

MEETING THE DEMANDS OF A DIVERSE POPULATION

One of the keys to chronic disease management is to target the right services to the right people. Within the average primary health care practice, most patients—perhaps two-thirds—do not currently have a major chronic medical condition, although many will be at future risk depending on both inherited and environmental factors. These individuals typically have little interaction with the health care system from year to year, other than routine visits with the primary care provider. With the right supports, these patients can be successful in managing their own care, reducing their future risks, and sustaining their own health. A significant portion could benefit from improved understanding of and support for healthy behaviours, including weight management, exercise, and tobacco cessation. For this group, the population health focus should be on engaging them in *self-management*.

An intermediate group (about 20%) of individuals has one or more chronic conditions and requires proactive management and support of their care by a multidisciplinary professional team. This second subset includes those with gradually progressing chronic conditions but who are not undergoing or facing imminent, acute exacerbations. This group generally requires anticipatory *care management* that includes the use of health care professionals to proactively address specific care needs (e.g., making sure the individual adheres to a medication regimen). Much of this can be done effectively through well-designed targeted information with direct assistance from care professionals.

Finally, there is a small portion, typically estimated at between 5 and 6%, who use a great deal of health care services. Generally speaking, these high users are increasingly drawn from recognized populations with multiple chronic conditions. These individuals are sicker and often have more complex conditions that benefit from active *case management* and access to first-rate clinician skills. Medical crises for these chronic conditions often require providers to address patients' health needs with expensive and specialized resources.

EFFICIENT RESOURCE ALLOCATION USING CHRONIC DISEASE MANAGEMENT

The health needs of the population can be envisaged as a pyramid, with the foundation representing low risk and the tip representing high risk (Figure 2.1). Over time, the natural progression for individuals is to move sequentially

Figure 2.1
Kaiser Permanente Population Health Risk Pyramid

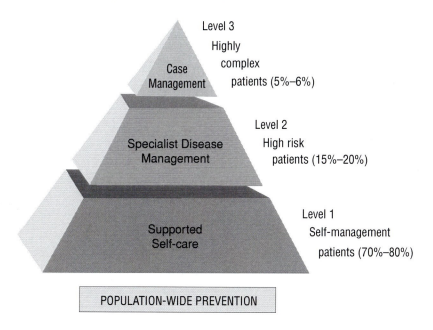

Note: Reprinted from *Chronic Disease Management: A Compendium of Information* (p. 17), by UK Department of Health, 2004, London: Department of Health Publications. Adapted from Kaiser Permanente.

up the pyramid. Therefore, the greatest challenge is to do what is necessary to prevent that upward migration associated with developing multiple and advanced chronic conditions. The economics of managing health risks over time are compelling, given the great cost savings to be gained from preventing moderate users from becoming intense consumers of expensive services. The larger and more immediate sources of return on investment lie in minimizing the need for sick care and improving the efficiency of case management. However, keeping the middle layer from ultimately requiring expensive hospital services (e.g., admissions for people with congestive heart failure) has both substantial quality and financial impacts.

For those responsible for allocating resources, the challenge often lies in determining where to focus resources and effort. The greatest benefit from resource investment derives from identifying those individuals at greatest risk of progressing up the population pyramid, as well as targeting likely acute events that are most amenable to prior interventions. That process involves three general steps.

- First, how does a provider identify those people at greatest *risk* for requiring acute care? Some conditions have more predictable determinants than others. Substantial advances have recently been made in the science of predictive modelling to help health plans and other organizations identify with increasing precision those at greatest risk.
- Second, once the highest risk population has been defined, the next question becomes: Is progression up the pyramid *amenable* to an upstream intervention that will decrease its likelihood of occurrence? For some chronic conditions, substantial research exists to guide health care teams as to the most effective approaches for managing care. Where research gaps exist, the expense of the acute event and/or the frequency of it in the population may still warrant concerted attempts to intervene with considerable resources.
- Third, consumers need to be *ready to change*. For most chronic conditions, successful care management depends to a considerable extent on the system's ability to engage the consumer as an active participant—if he or she has little interest in change, the investment of resources by the delivery system likely will yield little benefit.

The premise of chronic disease management is that we need to transform health care "from a system that is essentially reactive—responding mainly when a person is sick—to one that is proactive and focused on keeping a person as healthy as possible" (Improving Chronic Illness Care, 2007). Without targeted information prescribed to the individual at the right moment in care, consumers cannot be effectively engaged as partners in chronic disease management. Providing information to patients becomes a critical factor in supporting their ongoing involvement.

An additional critical factor in managing chronic condition care is to consider where to deliver care to be most effective. An individual with a chronic condition such as diabetes or heart failure will be confronted with at least some aspect of their care needs—diet, exercise, taking meds—24 hours a day, 7 days a week, 365 days a year. Of the 8,760 hours in a year, a patient will spend only a handful with his or her clinician or care team, while spending thousands of hours at work and around the home. Support for chronic conditions over this time frame does not need to be highly intense, but it does need to be consistently available, actionable, and persistent within the patient's daily routine.

For managing chronic conditions, an effective approach should involve at least three components:

- First, the approach must be durable over long periods of time when the individual (or patient) has little direct clinician contact. The individual's connection to the delivery system can certainly be enhanced by "virtual" contact, information prescriptions, and other forms of information exchange.
- Second, the approach needs to be effective in translating and disseminating evidence and knowledge from the system to the individual. This communication not only requires appropriate cataloging, structuring, and targeting of evidence-based information, but also requires translating it into a format that is both understandable and actionable by a population with a broad range of backgrounds and needs.
- Third, an effective chronic disease management approach needs to link to individual readiness to change. Different people respond to different methods at different times. The approach needs to be capable of preactivating the individual before a more focused contact with the health care delivery system is required (because that may be too late). This requires that the right information be prescribed at the right moment in care. By preactivating the patient, we can leverage the expensive act of that individual coming into the clinical office, thus maximizing the efficiency of the rest of the system.

The value proposition stretches even further because this transformation to chronic disease management coincides with a changing culture of consumer expectations. In the shifting environment, a chorus is growing with a mantra of "whatever I want, whenever I need it." Those health systems that fail to meet this evolving consumer demand face a serious potential opportunity cost. One can only expect that this set of consumer expectations will continue to grow in the years ahead.

The evidence is accumulating rapidly that engaging consumers in their own health management is a critical step toward fully achieving clinical goals of effective chronic disease management, but the benefits are more far-reaching than that. Returning to the population pyramid presented in Figure 2.1, it becomes clear that the economic benefits are potentially just as profound. Systems of care can achieve effective population care by using comparatively low-cost interventions broadly to prevent the migration of today's low utilizers into tomorrow's high utilizers. By effectively offering the right information at the right time, health care organizations can efficiently manage resources, as well. Importantly, net value will increase even if the absolute costs of care do not decrease (i.e., more value for the money spent), and evidence is growing that the use of chronic disease management is countering the trend of cost increases for the care of those with chronic conditions.

REFERENCES

Christopherson, G. (2004, September 27). *Ix Solutions Every Day: Person-Centered Care Via My HealtheVet/HealthePeople*. Presentation delivered at the Information Therapy Conference, Park City, Utah.

Improving Chronic Illness Care. (2007). *The Chronic Care Model*. Retrieved March 15, 2007, from http://www.improvingchroniccare.org/change/index.html

3. CHRONIC DISEASE MANAGEMENT—PLUS

Art Macgregor

MESH HEADINGS
British Columbia
Chronic disease
Depression
Diabetes mellitus
Disease management
Heart failure, congestive
Models, organizational
Quality assurance, health care

BACKGROUND

Recognition of the importance of chronic disease management and the role of primary medical care in health care in Canada is critical. Initiatives such as those stimulated by the federal Primary Health Care Transition Fund have provided added impetus to long overdue discussions on primary health care renewal and reform. That insights into the needs of both patients and caregivers should have to be "discovered" in the 21st century is remarkable. Despite this, many observers now agree that the role and potential of primary care has not been well understood, nor well supported, and that our primary medical care system in particular has been underperforming because of this lack of understanding and accompanying neglect of basic infrastructures needed for it to function up to its true potential.

This chapter outlines a Victoria, British Columbia, initiative in improving care of people with chronic conditions. It will emphasize an initial "ground-up" approach to quality improvement (QI), the historical evolution of a system-wide approach to QI, the local health care "culture," and the liberating and stimulating effect of a federal initiative in primary health care. It will include a discussion of the supports needed so that primary medical care can better contribute to the prevention of disease and the treatment of chronic conditions.

Necessity is indeed the mother of invention. In the early 1990s, the Victoria area was in danger of having a specialist shortage in endocrinology. The local family practice department then determined to improve its capability in diabetes care by an extensive series of Continuing Medical Education (CME) lectures with the expectation that family doctors might be able to look after a wider range of diabetic problems. This initiative was accompanied by a growing interest in QI by the local health authority, and the fortuitous timing of these activities led to a greater understanding of the complexity of improving services to patients. As primary care providers, we began to understand what has now become "obvious." One insight was that education alone does little to change physician behaviour; the other, much deeper, insight was that we all function interdependently within a system that has the capability of either nurturing high quality care or preventing it from happening. These insights did not come quickly or easily; they required investment in QI training such as participation in U.S.-based Institute for Healthcare Improvement (IHI) programs, further appreciation of the roles of many allied disciplines such as nursing and nutrition services, and formation of partnerships between practitioners and the health authority.

These combined activities led the Victoria group to take part in the first IHI collaborative in Canada, on Care of People With Chronic Conditions, in 1998–99. A team of four people (a family doctor, two nurses, and a dietitian) attended this year-long learning program and instituted a local change and improvement program focusing on diabetes, utilizing the offices and patients of 28 volunteer Victoria family doctors. The Chronic Care Model pioneered by Dr. Ed Wagner, national director of the Seattle-based MacColl Institute for Healthcare Innovation, was the organizing construct that we tried to emulate in a Canadianized version in our local health care system. It was from this experience that we began to understand that the Chronic Care Model provided a template to guide management of any and all chronic diseases. And we adopted Dr. Wagner's maxim that "the home of good chronic disease management lies in an enlightened primary care system." This insight has been very valuable in making us understand that family practice renewal and reform, and chronic disease management, are inextricably linked, and that any attempt to deal with them separately suggests a basic misunderstanding of how (and where) our health care system actually operates.

While all experts and guidelines extol the virtues of team care, and while everyone "knows" that one cannot deliver high quality care without adequate information systems, the reality in most parts of Canada, and certainly in British Columbia, has been that these vital infrastructures are largely missing in physician practices. It is not the purpose of this chapter to try to explain why this is so; most observers understand health care systems in Canada well enough to acknowledge that we are only now entering a time when governments and medical agencies are searching for ways to improve infrastructure, to deal with recruitment and retention problems in family practice and, at the same time, to improve care of people with chronic conditions. It comes then as no surprise to learn that the primary medical care system as we have known it has been ill-prepared to deliver comprehensive, continuing care for people with chronic conditions (see Table 3.1). Using the well-known diabetes model

Table 3.1
The Gap Between Needs and Services for Chronic Illnesses

What we think people with chronic conditions need:	*What they often get in Canada (despite many pockets of excellence):*
• long-term, trusting relationships with a small group of people	• short-term, episodic care from people they may not know and who may not know them
• consistent, competent, comprehensive services	• inconsistent, incomplete services
• convenient, readily accessible services	• delays and inaccessible services
• good quality, secure health records	• minimal records, often missing when needed
• partnerships, and nourishment of self-management capability	• increased anxiety, and decreased confidence in the health care system

(the canary in the chronic disease mine), we found that monitoring tests such as A1C, blood pressure, and lipids have been performed at about 40% of guideline-recommended rates. Canadian data for hypertension control have also shown this general pattern.

Our own experience in Victoria suggested, however, that very modest improvements in support could result in significant initial improvements in performance. In the 1998–99 project, testing rates for the three major parameters of diabetes management improved from the 40% zone to nearly double. No one imagined that this short-term volunteer project could of itself result in sustained improvements; relatively little in the way of system change actually happened. There was no immediate increase in incentive payment, no improvement in office IT capability, no provision of on-site multidisciplinary staff, and so forth. It did, however, suggest that there is a latent and powerful desire for change and improvement, that peer-led programs can have an impact, and that focused education that recognizes the real needs of doctors and patients can be very productive. What was missing in our earlier project was larger, supportive system changes. The emergence of the federal Primary Health Care Transition Fund (PHCTF) in 2000 helped to remedy this deficiency (temporarily) and, remarkably, stimulated changes in the whole British Columbia health care system.

HEALTH CARE "CLIMATE AND CULTURE" IN BRITISH
COLUMBIA IN 2003

Despite the presence in British Columbia of adequate numbers of family practitioners (on paper), the reality has been that doctors generally were dissatisfied
with many aspects of their professional lives. Many felt undervalued and
underremunerated compared to specialists and, indeed, to some other health
care workers. They felt that lip service had been paid to primary care being
the so-called backbone of the Canadian health care system. Some chaffed at
the idea that we needed to be "reformed" when many critics had been silent or
ineffective about the need for infrastructure support for doctors to do their
jobs. Team care seemed a distant dream for many who wondered who was
going to pay for all the salaries and other costs of the full team. In brief,
rightly or wrongly, many family doctors would not recommend the career to
their sons or daughters, and most new residency graduates seemed to be turn-
ing their attention to "anything but" full-service family practice. The effect of
all this seemed to explain, in part at least, the 40% performance rate in monitoring many chronic conditions as well as the growing number of "orphan
patients." From our earlier experience in the collaborative, we were aware
that family practice renewal and reform and good chronic disease management are inextricably linked, and that efforts to improve both professional
satisfaction and patient care might be focused on a QI initiative that seemed
to have the interests of both parties in mind.

A typical medical practice in Victoria, in 2003, might look something like
this: 1,200 patients, of whom about 50 have major depressive disorder, 50
have diabetes, 75 have chronic kidney disease, 100 have hypertension, and
100 have arthritis. Clearly, chronic disease management is about half of the
family doctor's routine work. In British Columbia, the realization that much
of our frustration and even burnout as family physicians can be blamed on the
mismatch between our job description and the support and incentives provided has had a powerful effect on medico-political discussions, fee
negotiations, and career choices of young physicians. The "TIC"—time, in-
tensity, and complexity of modern family practice—is now well understood.
The arrival of PHCTF funding for renewal activity, especially in the area of
Chronic Disease Management (CDM), was therefore particularly timely.

THE EXPANDED CHRONIC CARE MODEL

On June 18, 2003, we initiated a 3-year project using PHCTF funding (initially $2.1 million) entitled Implementing the Expanded Chronic Care Model
in an Integrated Primary Care System. Based on Wagner's Chronic Care Model,
this expanded version was revised to fit the Canadian approach to health care,
with an emphasis on the importance of the determinants of health. The model
is designed to assist in the care of an individual patient over time and also to
describe the care of a population of patients in a practice or community. From

the practitioner's point of view, four elements are critical (see the Health System components, Figure 3.1). The first and most urgent is an information system that describes the population at risk (e.g., the diabetes registry), and provides timely information about the current status of the patient according to guideline parameters. Our project developed an interim, web-based information system to get started; this was taken up by the provincial Ministry of Health and developed into what is now known as the CDM Toolkit. Utilizing this system, 30 family physicians joined the first wave of the project and developed registries for three chronic conditions: diabetes, congestive heart failure, and major depressive disorder. The electronic Toolkit allowed us to input monitoring data daily and to use recall and many other helpful reports to do self-audits and to improve practice. The second key element, delivery system redesign, encouraged an expanded scope of medical office assistant activity, the introduction of a small number of nurses and dietitians into physician offices to trial multidisciplinary care, and experimentation with group visits. Thirdly, decision support tools were vital; guidelines and flow sheets were used as basic reference points to guide daily work. Finally, and most crucially, genuine efforts were made to nurture patient self-management capability so that true partnerships between practitioners and patients might become a reality.

Figure 3.1
The Expanded Chronic Care Model

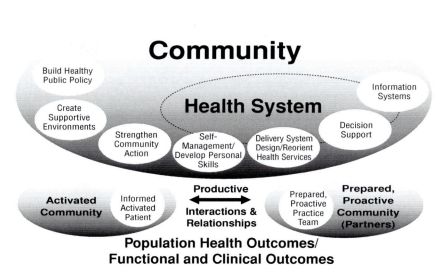

Note: Reprinted from "The Expanded Chronic Care Model: An Integration of Concepts and Strategies from Population Health Promotion and the Chronic Care Model," by V.J. Barr, S. Robinson, B. Marin-Link, L. Underhill, A. Dotts, and D. Ravensdale, 2003, *Healthcare Quarterly, 7*(1), pp. 73-82.

The initial success of this project was recognized in 2004 with 3M Canada's Health Care Quality Team Award, which stimulated further funding and recruitment. In the last year of the project, the group participated in the provincial Prevention Support Program (see chapter 6). Seventeen physicians also attempted to integrate preventive medicine approaches with their patients in the 50 to 70 age group. A total of 10,000 patients were directly impacted by these QI initiatives (approximately 6,500 with chronic conditions and 3,500 in the prevention arm).

This project was an attempt to implement best known current practice in the offices of conventional fee-for-service physicians, and in a small number of salaried physicians' offices. We were guided in this attempt by the following principles and strategies:

1. Implement a well-tested, comprehensive model of care which takes into account all patient and practice issues that impact daily care.
2. Illustrate the first law of QI as succinctly stated by Donald Berwick, president and CEO of IHI: "Every system is perfectly designed to produce the results it gets." Instead of blaming anyone for a 40% performance rate, we would look to system issues and attempt to understand them, alter them where possible, and lobby where appropriate for system-wide change.
3. Use the IHI collaborative learning model and exploit the powerful effect of a collaborative of doctors, nurses, dietitians, and others coming together regularly to improve their mutual abilities to help people.
4. Provide incentives for physicians to do some of the "extra" things not provided for in the current fee system (e.g., regular data input, data analysis, attendance at meetings, and modest assistance with IT).
5. Improve professional satisfaction in practice by enhancing support systems and the capacity of primary care workers, and by showing that we have the power within our group to influence the local health care system.

An open appeal to all local physicians to join a CDM-QI collaborative was over-subscribed; 30 were originally selected. An attempt was made to balance solo and group practices, and younger and older physicians, and to have a representative community-wide group. Two RNs, a data analyst, a part-time project manager, and medical leads were hired. A logic model outlining the project's origins, goals, and strategies was created. Three common diseases—diabetes, congestive heart failure, and major depressive disorder—were selected in order to show that the Expanded Chronic Care Model is in fact generic in nature and can be used to guide the prevention and management of any chronic condition. IHI-style learning sessions were held every 3 months from June 2003 to March 2006. Project staff, in particular the RNs, were important in facilitating registry development, as was IT support from the provincial Ministry of Health. Registries of the three conditions were created, new provincial guidelines for these conditions fortuitously appeared at the same time, flow sheets were developed in conjunction with a conjoint Ministry/British Columbia Medical Association committee, and disease-specific data collection using the web-based system began. In addition to disease-specific data elements, general care considerations such as efforts to nurture self-management were documented. Instruction in retrieving reports from the information system was given, and at quarterly meetings our data analyst prepared doctor-specific and comparative collaborative data to assess progress. Feedback to physicians was intended to be confidential, but we soon discovered that in a supportive QI atmosphere a great deal of data sharing occurred that helped both in fostering a competitive spirit and mutuality in the sharing of learning experiences.

With increasing evidence of improvement in outcomes, we were able to attract more funding and more participants in successive waves. A total of 65 physicians, 4 nurses, and 1 dietitian ultimately participated. Of great interest was the opportunity to add a preventive medicine component to the CDM project in the last year. The ability of physicians to integrate preventive medicine easily into routine practice was very instructive again in illustrating the simple point that QI changes can be produced by very modest incentives if accompanied by supportive staff and an environment that fosters change.

OUTCOMES

Two types of measures were used to track outcomes. The first measure, *processes of care*, included the use of appropriate and specific diagnostic tests (e.g., echocardiography for congestive heart failure and PHQ-9 for depression), monitoring (e.g., A1C, blood pressure, and lipids for diabetes), guideline-recommended prescribing (e.g., ACE inhibitors for systolic heart failure), and use of appropriate patient-centred aids such as self-management visits. A second type of measurement involved (surrogate) *outcomes of care* such as actual lab values (e.g., A1C, lipid tests, and proportion at goal). All of these outcomes were available to individual participants directly from the Toolkit reports and, in addition, were analyzed in detail at a collaborative level at quarterly meetings.

Table 3.2 is a summary of some of the outcomes tracked in the program. It should be noted that this project was an implementation project, not a research project. The aim was to implement best known practice in the offices of family practitioners, and to collect data during or shortly after the clinical encounter. Physician and staff data input could not be subjected to rigorous data quality control. Table 3.2 represents our best estimates of actual performance.

Of those diabetic patients that had all three tests done, those complying with Canadian Diabetes Association guidelines improved from 21.8% to 48.6% over the project period. It should also be noted that some of the "start" rates and values were higher than provincial averages due to earlier QI work in the Victoria area.

LESSONS LEARNED

There is no doubt that a number of events fortuitously occurred in our region to facilitate this project. As was noted, a supportive local health authority

Table 3.2
Outcomes of the BC Chronic Disease Management Programs

Programs	Testing June 2003 (Baseline %)	Testing February 2006 (%)	% Meeting Guideline Goals February 2006
Diabetes			
A1C	66.2	79.1	72.8
Blood pressure	63.9	73.2	74.0
Lipids	54.0	74.5	70.1
Microalbumin	41.5	70.0	n/a
Congestive heart failure			
ACE/ARB (prescribed)	60.2	85.7	
Beta-blocker (Syst) (prescribed)	31.6	72.4	
Depression			
PHQ-9	9.0	46.0	

Note: The A1C test measures long-term blood sugar control. ACE/ARB = angiotensin converting enzyme inhibitor or angiotensin II receptor blocker. PHQ-9 is a patient health questionnaire that assesses depression on a 9-item scale.

initiated training in QI, which gave many staff, including some local family physicians, an opportunity to participate directly in an IHI collaborative. This early diabetes improvement project gave us experience and confidence and provided a ready model to be expanded by the use of the federal funds. The leadership role of physician champions, and the willingness of the local health authority and Ministry to partner in constructive ways were key. The important role of inspirational project managers and the skilled facilitation of the collaborative's work by nurses and a dietitian should be emphasized. This was the first experience for many in implementing the team concept in health care delivery. Finally, it must be recognized that there was an underlying demand on the part of physicians for some constructive way to improve their ability to care for people and to receive greater recognition for and professional satisfaction from their sometimes undervalued but important work.

Other lessons learned include the following:

- A modest investment in the primary care worker will yield enormous payoffs.
- The need for improved information systems in health care has been made crystal clear; however, the cost and complexities of this improvement are significant.
- There are real difficulties in instituting shared care with specialists, with the exception of mental health specialists, who have a different experience and funding system. Shared care with other specialities will require a great deal more study and investment.

- The opportunity to work with allied health professionals has been welcomed by many in our group of family physicians. Those who had experience with on-site nursing and dietitian support wanted more. The difficulty, however, is funding this team concept.
- Despite a great deal of physician education in nurturing patient self-management, we have found that this "simple" idea is not easy to implement. While most physicians believe that they have always encouraged self-management, in practice many issues interfere. Time for discussion is in short supply. Further, the conventional medical approach of looking for what is "wrong" is an initial barrier to self-management, which involves strengthening what is "right" with the patient.
- Guidelines are only guidelines! They need a realistic implementation plan to go with them and they need frequent revision.
- There is a limit to improvement—a "ceiling." In our particular context, it appears to be about 80%. Much more in the way of system change will be needed to get to the 90%–100% performance level.
- It is critically important to understand system issues, such as incentives and infrastructure supports, and their relation to desired health care outcomes. Instruction to develop group practices with no consideration of the expense and complexities (e.g., real estate and IT issues) is a losing strategy.
- Finally, a powerful lesson to us is how influential a community collaborative can be in influencing public policy. The Expanded Chronic Care Model is now well-known in the province, and recent fee negotiations have been positively influenced by the experience of collaboratives in CDM. Greater understanding and respect for partnerships between providers and funders is now much more evident, and CDM initiatives appear to be an unusually good lever with which to engage physicians and governments.

QI seems to require some kind of change. Since few people want to be changed (especially by governments), it is clear that a key success factor is to offer change and improvement opportunities that appeal to the personal, social, or professional interests of physicians. Appropriate incentives and opportunities to be equal partners with other health care workers and with regional and provincial governments are critical. Organized collaboratives are one, but only one, vehicle for change. What must now happen is for lessons learned in British Columbia cooperatives and positive experiences in several other provinces to be applied more widely and much more quickly. Neither the public, nor government, nor practitioners have patience for delay; much is now known, much remains to be done. The test now is whether or not there is the imagination or will to institute some of these obvious improvements on a large scale.

4. CHRONIC DISEASE MANAGEMENT IN A COMPREHENSIVE, INTEGRATED PRIMARY CARE SETTING

David Crookston and Elizabeth Bodnar

MESH HEADINGS
Chronic disease
Diabetes mellitus
Disease management
Heart failure, congestive
Medical records systems, computerized
Ontario
Patient care team
Primary health care

BACKGROUND

Group Health Centre (GHC) of Sault Ste. Marie, Ontario, is Canada's first consumer-sponsored, prepaid medical program. It was built on a foundation of unique principles, including a group medical practice, consumer sponsorship, and prepayment of medical insurance—very innovative ideas in 1962. The momentum for the Centre began in the late 1950s, with union leaders who carried the new idea to the workplace and the community. These visionaries canvassed for funds in subzero weather, convincing 5,000 union members to give $135 each, for a total of over $675,000 to build the Centre (About GHC, Our History section, 2007). Today, GHC is a multispecialty, interdisciplinary, ambulatory care facility with diagnostic services and electronic medical records. As Ontario's largest and oldest membership-based health care organization, it provides health care services to most of the population in Sault Ste. Marie and the surrounding District of Algoma.

A joint management committee, with equal representation from the boards of the Group Health Association (GHA) and the Algoma District Medical Group (ADMG), recommends planning decisions. The success of the GHC is fundamentally dependent upon the willing cooperation between the independent medical group (ADMG) and the independent not-for-profit corporation (GHA).

The Centre was initially built to secure health care services in a community struggling with a shortage of health care providers, which is very similar to today's health care human-resource challenges. This model of care was designed to ensure that patients receive the right care, at the right time, by the most appropriate provider. GHC's philosophy is to promote health and prevent illness, provide better health outcomes, prevent or reduce hospital admissions, and encourage patient education and self-care. Its programs and services have developed over the years to become a model of primary care excellence, supporting a network of chronic disease programs through the use of an interdisciplinary team approach and innovative information technology.

GHC originally opened with 13 physicians and 35 staff providing care for 12,000 patients. As of 2006, it has 61 physicians and associates, and over 300 allied professionals and staff providing services to a rostered population of more than 60,000 patients. At its inception, the diligence and strong leadership of the founding members, combined with the willingness of a group of physicians to practice in a setting that had not yet received the general approval of organized medicine, permitted an idea to grow into reality. The development of interdisciplinary teams using medical directives, with a focus on maximizing scope of practice, was a necessary shift from independent medical practice. In order to work in this environment, a culture shift was necessary. As the model developed and grew, strong leadership and cooperation between the two partnerships, the GHA and the ADMG, were necessary components of the organization's success.

In 1997, a key decision to implement an Electronic Medical Records (EMR) system was unanimously supported by both boards. This decision was critical in transforming the delivery of care for GHC patients by providing a common platform for sharing information and care plans among physicians and allied health professionals. The implementation of this system—Canada's largest primary care EMR—and the subsequent transition from paper-based charts, was very challenging, but it has become the cornerstone of GHC's evidence-based, chronic disease management and research programs. It is used by all providers—every physician and allied provider at the Centre. This "paperless" environment tracks all clinical activity on a patient, including visits to physicians (primary and specialty), allied providers, clinics, labs, hospitals, and so forth, thus creating one of the most comprehensive records available. A strong information technology (IT) infrastructure is critical, but information technologists must have a good understanding of physician flow and processes. Identifying the impact of IT on medical staff should include context, workflow, finances, and culture.

With strong community and government support, the GHC model can be applied to the broader health care system. Currently, some aspects of the Family Health Teams being established in Ontario are being patterned after the GHC model. Hopefully, this will enable the development of integrated chronic disease management programs to ensure that the growing population of "baby boomers" requiring additional care in the coming years will be able to access that care through interdisciplinary teams using electronic medical records.

One of the Centre's most outstanding programs, established to prevent and manage chronic disease, is the Health Promotion Initiatives (HPI) program, a partnership of GHC providers. Under the direction of the joint management committee, the HPI team, made up of several physicians and managers, meets once a month to administer the program. The HPI concept was created by Dr. Hui Lee, who died tragically in 2004. Hui was an inspiration to those who were fortunate enough to practice, work with, and know him. His HPI legacy continues to grow as a tribute to his brilliance and dedication.

HPI was created to develop and evaluate evidence-based, outcomes-management programs and to improve the quality of health care for GHC's 60,000 rostered patients. Disease site registries have been developed through the use of IT systems including electronic medical records, practice management applications, and web technology. What began as an innovative idea is now a network of quality management and improvement programs that demonstrates our accountability to patients, providers, and funders.

Active programs in diabetes, congestive heart failure, anticoagulation, osteoporosis, smoking cessation, immunization, asthma, and cervical and mammography screening have been established and continue to enable improved patient outcomes. Projects in the development stage are vascular intervention, chronic obstructive pulmonary disease, and mental health. GHC is also looking to use IT to advance the management of chronic disease through the enhanced sharing of clinical information between community physicians, pharmacists, and patients. Currently, physicians and pharmacists in the community are still working in silos with no direct connectivity and means of collaboration for sharing clinical information. Including the community pharmacist in the circle of care through the EMR would break down these silos.

Some unique and innovative aspects of the HPI program are its

- focus on population health and primary care delivery in an interdisciplinary setting;
- chronic disease management infrastructure, including patient and health care provider education;
- close collaboration with other academic and health care organizations;
- application of continuous quality improvement principles; and
- common platform (EMR) for sharing information and care plans among all health care providers.

The Health Promotion Initiatives program is innovative in its structure. The interdisciplinary team approach, with clinical leadership, is supported by an electronic medical record that facilitates communication among team members and the monitoring of patient outcomes. In addition, the interdisciplinary team is supported by medical directives, which maximize scope of practice.

In March 2004 the Ministry of Health and Long-Term Care awarded Primary Health Care Transition Funding to GHC to conduct a Vascular Intervention Project (VIP) under our HPI programs. Results of this study will be available in 2007. The VIP has two key components. The first is the reduction of vascular risk through the utilization of an ACTION score, a self-management tool that responds to the patient's lifestyle and other interventions to reduce his or her modifiable risk factors. The second component is the development of VIPNet, a patient portal on GHC's website that enables patients to become more involved in self-managing their care, and to share their health status with other members within the circle of care.

OUTCOMES

Our HPI success is measured in improved health outcomes for our patients, which are identified in the following examples:

- A nurse-run anticoagulation clinic to monitor patient International Normalized Ratios (INRs) has become the largest clinic of its kind in Canada, with 583 patients. Through the use of clinical leadership and medical directives, 3 years of data show that 84% of GHC INRs are in therapeutic range (+/–0.2%), compared to "usual care" benchmarks in the 40%–60% range. Major bleeding events are rare (< 1%).
- A collaborative community program was developed to improve health outcomes for patients with Congestive Heart Failure (CHF). Figure 4.1 illustrates that the program initially achieved a 43% reduction in hospital readmission rates for this group of patients, which has been sustained over 5 years. These outstanding results, and information on our CHF program, are included in the Change Foundation's report, *Seeking Program Sustainability in Chronic Disease Management: The Ontario Experience* (Wong, Gilbert, & Kilburn, 2004).

Figure 4.1
Results of the Congestive Heart Failure (CHF) Pilot Program,
from January to June 2000

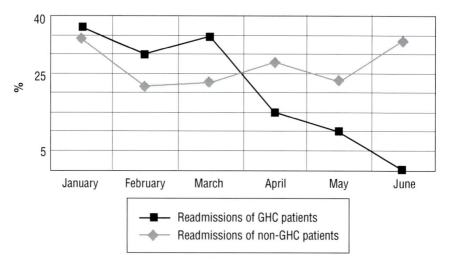

- The creation of the Algoma Breast Health Program, which is a collaborative effort of the Sault Area Hospital, GHC, and the Ontario Breast Screening Program, has successfully reduced wait times from breast cancer diagnosis to surgical intervention from 108 days to less than a month. In addition, 70.6% of female GHC patients received mammography screening, versus the national average of 53.6% based on the 1996/97 National Population Health Survey (Maxwell, Bancej, & Snider, 2001).
- Through a joint collaborative project with our local public health unit, our community flu clinics immunized 22,155 patients in 2005, a 7% increase over the previous year. This success is the result of strong community collaboration and the use of innovative systems to improve efficiencies in process. To vaccinate such a large number of patients in such a short period of time, we utilized an electronic patient appointment system to book patients into a flu clinic held in a local mall. Staff were extremely satisfied to be able to provide service without waits, in an environment that was very accessible for patients.
- GHC's Diabetes Program, which is open to community patients, currently provides education and care to 3,415 patients. The program has developed health outcome measurements based on the Canadian Diabetes Association's clinical practice guidelines. The HPI team developed a template within the EMR to support the care given to patients with diabetes. This tool enables primary care providers (general practitioners and nurse practitioners) to effectively monitor patients with diabetes and ensure timely, proactive treatment that meets best practice guidelines. In addition, primary care providers receive a summary of their Good Health Outcomes for Diabetes (GHOD) score, which measures 12 process and clinical outcomes. Figure 4.2 reflects outcome improvements for our diabetes patients over 5 years. For the entire diabetes population identified in the registry, the HbA1C control improved from 44.6% to 53.45% between 2000 and 2005, about a 9% increase. However, for patients who accessed the Diabetes Program, the implementation of medical directives for insulin and oral diabetes medication adjustment improved HbA1C by an impressive 20% from 42.4% to 62%.
- We have been successful in knowledge transfer in many ways, including participation in a number of national health care best practice showcases, invitational lectures, and policy advisory committees.

LESSONS LEARNED

HPI developed from a concept to an established program that is integral to primary care excellence at GHC. Chronic disease management is a challenge in today's health care system, where financial resources are limited and the community is boxed into silos of care. Strong leadership at a governance and clinical level was necessary not only to establish the program, but to deal with ongoing challenges such as maintaining enthusiasm in the face of personnel shortages and conflicting demands, finding common ground in partnerships,

Figure 4.2
Five-Year Outcomes of the Health Promotion Initiatives (HPI) Diabetes Program

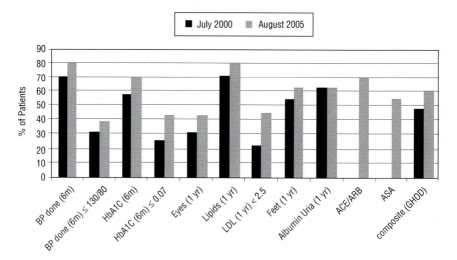

Note: BP = blood pressure. HbA1C is a hemoglobin test that measures blood sugar. LDL = low density lipoprotein. ACE/ARB = angiotensin converting enzyme inhibitor or angiotensin II receptor blocker. ASA = acetylsalicylic acid. GHOD = Good Health Outcomes for Diabetes.

responding to evolving standards (the bar keeps moving), balancing sick care with chronic disease management, and coping with change fatigue. Without strong financial and corporate leadership, the implementation of the HPI program would not have been successful.

Continuous assessment and evaluation, using an EMR, is another key to success. The principles of HPI aid the provision of appropriate, evidence-based care because guidelines by themselves do not work. The implementation of an EMR and the transition from a paper-based chart to an electronic chart was a huge culture and system change that has enabled the development of the HPI programs.

An interdisciplinary team is essential to support these initiatives. By sharing the same vision and maximizing the scope of practice, team members create a positive momentum and acknowledge everyone's effort. In addition, the team members improve their own performance through a sharing of knowledge, the learning process, and the support of other team members. The development of interdisciplinary teams with a focus on maximizing scope of practice and using medical directives was a necessary shift from independent practice that ensures the right care, at the right time, by the right provider.

The HPI program could be applied to other health care systems that support collaborative partnerships and the use of electronic databases. The key concepts of leadership, an interdisciplinary team approach, and the monitoring of health outcomes are basic for the application within other communities. GHC hosts visits from other health care providers across the country, who come to learn about our EMR, primary care delivery model, and chronic disease management programs. In addition, GHC is represented on the Family Health Team Action Group, which is assisting the Ontario government to transform the province's health care system. Not all systems need to be the same to be successful. However, the key concepts of the GHC program are necessary for implementation of chronic disease management in an integrated, primary care setting.

Here is some advice to other programs contemplating change:

- Look to the evidence and then start with small pilot projects and controlled trials. Measure the outcomes and, if successful, expand the project to the whole patient population.
- Maintain control over the process of managing the data. Show providers their own data and encourage them to join the project for improved outcomes.
- Show leadership with a broader, collaborative community approach, rather than focusing on your own organizational or individual gains. In doing this, consider forming partnerships with other private and public service providers. There is mutual advantage to sharing and collaborating with others who provide service in the same community.
- Keep the patient at the heart of the initiative. By involving patients and their families in the management of their care and by setting goals that improve patient health outcomes, you can monitor your success in patient care.

REFERENCES

Group Health Centre. (2007). About GHC, Our History section. Retrieved March 5, 2007, from http://www.ghc.on.ca/about/content.html?sID=84

Group Health Centre. (2007). VIPNet. Retrieved March 1, 2007, from http://www.ghc.on.ca/home.html

Maxwell, C.J., Bancej, C.M., & Snider, J. (2001). Predictors of mammography use among Canadian women aged 50–69: Findings from the 1996/97 National Population Heath Survey. *Canadian Medical Association Journal 164*(3), 329-33.

Wong, J., Gilbert, J., & Kilburn, L. (2004). *Seeking program sustainability in chronic disease management.* Retrieved February 20, 2007, from the Change Foundation website, http://www.changefoundation.com/tcf/TCFBul.nsf/(S001)/004E81ADB65E173C85256E940046509A

5. DEVELOPING CHRONIC DISEASE POLICY IN ENGLAND

Rebecca Rosen

MESH HEADINGS
Case management
Chronic disease
Disease management
Health care reform
Health policy
Models, organizational
Risk
Risk factors
Self-care
United Kingdom

BACKGROUND

The worldwide epidemic of chronic diseases is affecting England, and the English National Health Service (NHS), in the same way as many other countries. As the population ages, the number of people living with one or more chronic conditions is increasing. Historic smoking patterns underlie epidemics of respiratory and heart disease. A new epidemic of obesity is driving up the incidence of diabetes and further fuelling other chronic diseases. Over 1.3 million people in England have been diagnosed with diabetes, with up to 1 million more living with undiagnosed symptoms. Over 600,000 have chronic obstructive lung disease (COPD), around 8.5 million are living with arthritis, and up to one in six people are affected by mental health problems. Since 1997, policy to promote devolution of political control to the four countries of the UK—England, Scotland, Wales, and Northern Ireland—has resulted in a divergence in health policy between these countries. This chapter will describe English health policy on chronic diseases in the context of health system reform.

Chronic conditions drive a high proportion of inpatient hospital care and, thus, much of the cost of modern health care. Analysis of hospital admission data revealed that 50% of bed-day use is caused by 2.7% of conditions, and 25% of bed-day use is caused by 0.7% of conditions including COPD, heart disease, diabetes, depression and schizophrenia (see Figure 5.1). Most of these bed days arise from emergency admissions due to a critical deterioration in

Figure 5.1
Cumulative Bed-Day Use by ICD Code

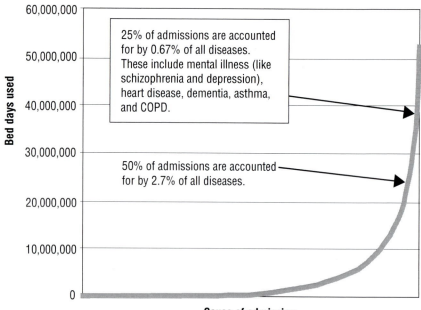

Note: ICD = International Classification of Diseases. COPD = chronic obstructive pulmonary disease. Reprinted from *Chronic Disease Management: A Compendium of Information* (p. 9), by UK Department of Health, 2004, London: Department of Health Publications. Copyright 2004 by Crown Copyright.

clinical symptoms, yet there is good evidence that many admissions could be avoided with better primary and community care.

England has a long tradition of chronic disease management, dating back to policy papers in the 1980s from the Royal College of General Practitioners (1981) advocating the use of disease registers and organized care for people with chronic diseases. In 1990 a new national contract for general practitioners (GPs) included payments to run chronic disease clinics. In the late 1990s the burden of preventable illness and premature death caused by heart disease and mental health problems was the focus of key public health targets in the government's White Paper, *Saving Lives: Our Healthier Nation* (Department of Health, 1999b).

There is also a long tradition of case management organized by social services departments. Social services (social workers, home helps, residential care services, etc.) in England are funded and provided by (elected) local governments, while health services are provided by (unelected) NHS health authorities. Since the mid-1980s, there have been initiatives to reduce the need for, and cost of, long-stay residential and nursing home care through the co-ordinated planning and provision of intensive social care support—that is, case management—for frail older people with complex needs. The philosophy and approach of case management (a coordinated, planned, proactive approach combining assessment, care planning, care provision, monitoring progress, regular review, and reassessment) is thus well established among social care providers.

The drive to achieve the targets in *Saving Lives:Our Healthier Nation* (Department of Health, 1999b) is being supported by of a series of *National Service Frameworks* (NSFs). Produced by the Department of Health, these reports are evidence-based, national blueprints for the effective delivery of health services for specific conditions (e.g., mental health, heart disease, diabetes [1999a, 2000, 2002]), care groups (e.g., older people [2001]), and children's services (2004a). They outline the range of services—covering prevention, diagnosis, treatment and, where appropriate, palliation—that should be provided and set standards for the quality of care expected across the whole country.

With explicit timetables and reporting mechanisms linked to their implementation, the NSFs were both impressive and problematic. They triggered much activity to improve services, but they also drove people to work in silos. Diabetes services were developing in isolation from heart disease services despite the fact that many of the patients affected by the two conditions were the same.

By 2003 several factors had triggered a refocusing of English health policy. First, the Labour government believed it had "cracked" the NHS waiting list problem that for so had long fuelled politically damaging headlines. Since coming to power in 1997, the government had introduced a series of new policies to increase capacity in the NHS including employing more doctors and nurses and introducing private sector providers for planned surgeries in order to cut waiting lists. Second, awareness of the impact and cost of chronic disease in the NHS had grown to a level where it became a key policy priority. Third, research comparing the performance of the NHS to the U.S.-managed health care organization, Kaiser Permenante, had been published (Feachem, Sekhri, & White, 2002) suggesting that Kaiser achieved better value for money from its health services. This stimulated regular visits to Kaiser and other U.S.-managed care organizations, and allowed rapid learning about the systematic, proactive care that was being offered by some health plans (Dixon, Lewis, Rosen, Grey, & Finlayson, 2004) in line with the Chronic Care Model (Wagner, 1998).

The results, in policy terms, of this period of rapid international learning and home-based reflection on the strengths and weaknesses of NSFs are discussed below after a brief consideration of the context and terminology of English policy on long-term conditions.

HIGH-LEVEL POLICY CONTEXT

It is hard to understand the impact of recent English policy on long-term conditions without understanding the wider policy context in which it has been introduced. The NHS is a huge state bureaucracy, employing over 1 million people, tightly managed by central government and accountable to parliament through the Secretary of State for Health. Despite the efforts of numerous health ministers to cut waiting lists, increase efficiency, and improve services, the pace of change in the NHS has often been painfully slow with areas of innovation and excellence matched by areas of inertia and out-of-date practice.

Little changed for three years after the Labour government came to power in 1997, but in 2000 it launched a comprehensive plan to modernize the NHS. *The NHS Plan* (Department of Health, 2004b), and a series of policies that have followed, aspired to offer NHS patients (for whom tax funding supports a comprehensive service, free at the point of delivery with a small, fixed copayment for drugs) a level of choice and service quality similar to what is available to those with (entirely optional) private medical insurance.

The policies also reflected a new philosophical approach to the NHS—the need for choice and competition to drive change, and for increased responsiveness to patients and overall efficiency. Historically, the NHS was both *funded* and *provided* by the state. Thus, NHS hospitals were state owned, and doctors, nurses and other health professionals were all state employees. Funding flowed from central government to local health authorities, to hospitals and GPs via a complicated set of formulas and contracts that have never fully matched payment to the cost of care provided. The district general hospital serving a particular area is part of the fabric of the local community and seen by the public as "our" hospital. In addition, a small amount of NHS care has always been provided by private hospitals—mainly through fee-for-service contracts for planned operations in order to reduce waiting lists. An overview of recent major NHS reforms is presented in Figure 5.2.

Figure 5.2
Overview of National Health Service (NHS) System Reform

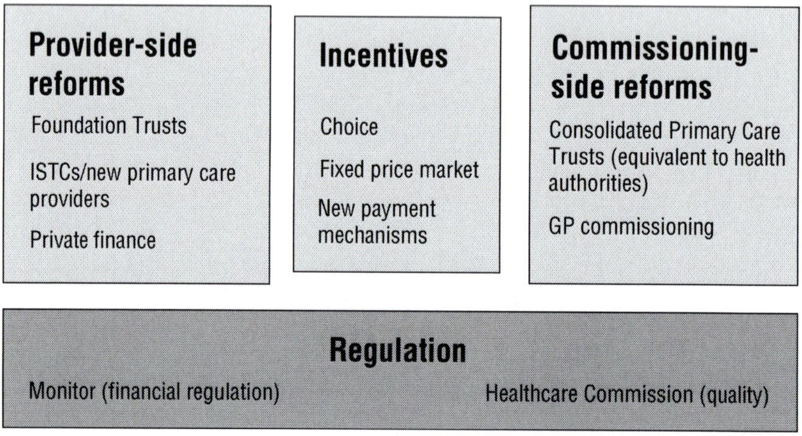

Provider-side reforms	**Incentives**	**Commissioning-side reforms**
Foundation Trusts	Choice	Consolidated Primary Care Trusts (equivalent to health authorities)
ISTCs/new primary care providers	Fixed price market	
Private finance	New payment mechanisms	GP commissioning

Regulation	
Monitor (financial regulation)	Healthcare Commission (quality)

Note: ISTC = Independent Sector Treatment Centre. The ISTC program is part of an NHS initiative to create additional capacity by reducing wait times and introducing choice for patients. GP = general practitioner.

The new organizing principle of the NHS centres around markets and competition. Current policy is based on the belief that it should not matter who provides health care to NHS patients as long as it is provided at a price set by the NHS (the national tariff price), is of high quality, and free at the point of delivery. *The NHS Plan* heralded the introduction of private providers of health care to compete with NHS hospitals for up to 15% of planned operations in the first instance. Subsequent policy has signalled that much more private provision is likely in other parts of the health service including primary care and chronic disease management. Some of the key mechanisms to achieve these policy goals are as follows:

- *Payment by results* This new payment system reimburses hospitals for each procedure or episode of care provided. Payment is at a national fixed rate— the tariff—which reflects the national average cost for that intervention, adjusted for certain local market forces. Payment by results effectively offers hospitals a fee-for-service payment for each episode of care, incentivizing additional interventions (desirable in relation to planned surgery in order to keep waiting lists down) and penalizing reduced activity (desirable in relation to better care for long-term conditions, where hospitalization can be seen as a failure to stay well).
- *Patient choice* Patients are allowed to choose between a cluster of different hospitals (or other care providers) when their GP refers them for specialist care. Although patients used to be able to choose freely between NHS hospitals, choice has been much more limited since the early 1990s. Early studies have shown that, when offered the choice, some people express a willingness to travel to distant hospitals if they can have a planned operation more quickly. However, such choices are less relevant to people with long-term conditions, many of whom are elderly with multiple diagnoses and require regular hospital visits.
- *Foundation trusts* Some NHS hospitals have been granted a quasi-independent status that frees them from direct accountability to the Secretary of State. The rules of the NHS bureaucracy were seen as a potential constraint on the ability of NHS hospitals to compete fairly with new private providers, so the best NHS hospitals have been granted a form of "earned autonomy." The status gives them certain organizational and financial freedoms, such as the ability to depart from national pay rates and develop their own investment plans. Foundation trusts are accountable to an independent regulator, and hospitals are only granted foundation status after careful scrutiny of their financial and organizational "fitness" (Lewis, 2005).
- *Independent sector health care providers* First announced in *The NHS Plan* in relation to planned surgery, subsequent policy has signalled the likely growth of private provision to NHS patients. The 2006 White Paper, *Our Health, Our Care, Our Say* (Department of Health, 2006a), indicates that private providers will be encouraged to provide primary care services in selected areas and to offer disease management and telehealth services.

These key areas of health policy in 2006 create both opportunities and threats to policy on long-term conditions. The Chronic Care Model argues that high quality care requires evidence-based care pathways spanning clinical and community settings. This care is best provided through partnerships and teamwork among general practitioners, specialist nurses, hospital specialists, therapists, and others. But the incentives inherent in current policy encourage more hospital activity rather than less and may well disrupt the relationships required between community and hospital practitioners. These points will be revisited in the discussion section below.

LONG-TERM CONDITIONS POLICY, 2004–2005

From the start, policy makers recognized that people with chronic diseases manage their conditions mostly themselves. These patients have contact with health professionals for only a few hours a year, and rely largely on their own skills, caregivers, support groups, and patient organizations to try to stay well. Patient organizations such as Diabetes UK were invited to participate in policy-making groups and quickly formed into an organized group to represent the voices of the estimated 17 million people living with chronic diseases (17 Million Reasons, 2005). Their first contribution to the policy debate was to condemn use of the term *chronic diseases*. They argued that people do not understand what chronic means, and those living with conditions such as depression or anxiety do not have a disease. The term *long-term conditions*, they believe, captures more fairly the experience of *all* those to whom policy should be targeted. This term is now used in key English policy documents.

A substantial body of policy has been developed on long-term conditions since 2004. The policy is predicated on two models for providing care to this large and diverse group of patients:

1. The first is the well-known Chronic Care Model, developed by Wagner (1998) and his colleagues at the MacColl Institute for Healthcare Innovation in Seattle, Washington (see chapter 1).
2. The second is a risk pyramid developed by Kaiser Permenante in California (see chapter 2, Figure 2.1) that depicts the population living with long-term conditions in three broad groups. Approximately 3%–5% of people at the top of the pyramid are considered to be at high risk of clinical deterioration and hospital admission. These people are typically older, and are living with several long-term conditions.

Recognizing that people with complex long-term conditions often need social support as well as health services, recent policy has emphasized the need for integration between health and social care. The key policy document on long-term conditions, *Supporting People with Long-Term Conditions* (Department of Health, 2005b), emphasized three important policy directions: case management, disease management, and self-management.

CASE MANAGEMENT

In early 2004, the Department of Health announced that it would fund pilot sites of the Evercare model of nurse-led case management developed by United Health Care in America. A cadre of highly skilled "advanced nurse practitioners" would be developed to provide intensive, clinically focused case management for people over 65 years at high risk of hospitalization. The Evercare pilots were established in 10 Primary Care Trusts (PCTs)—local health boards that commission health services for populations of approximately 150,000 to 200,000—and were expected to reduce hospital admissions in this group by up to 50%.

Although a rigorous evaluation was commissioned from a leading UK research centre, policy on nurse-led case management was rolled out long before the results were available. In mid-2004, the Department of Health announced that 3,000 "community matrons" would be trained across the country to case manage people with complex long-term conditions, coordinate care across settings, advocate for their needs, and support them to self-manage their problems. Community matrons were seen as a central part of the Department's response to its 2004 Public Service Agreement with the treasury (which ultimately funds the health service) to reduce the number of emergency bed days used by NHS patients by 5% by 2008.

There was widespread confusion at the local level about what exactly community matrons were—the PR-conscious government was keen on buzzwords and thought the public would like the idea of a "matron." There were also many questions about where the community matrons would come from in an already depleted nursing workforce, how they could develop the necessary skills, and how they would be funded. However, their role was gradually clarified (see Figure 5.3) and by 2006 the majority of PCTs had a cluster of community matrons working with high-risk patients with complex long-term conditions. Their impact on emergency hospital admissions remains unclear.

DISEASE MANAGEMENT

Disease management of specific conditions forms the second arm of long-term conditions policy. Building on progress with implementing NSFs, disease management focuses on single conditions. This disease-specific care may be provided to individuals who are living with only one condition, or to people with multiple conditions. Thus, high-risk patients may receive care from one or more specialist disease-management teams (such a community respiratory team and a heart-failure nurse specialist), in addition to care from a community matron who seeks to coordinate care from multiple providers.

There have been two key developments in disease management policy. First, the implementation of the NSFs, which predate recent policy on long-term conditions, have stimulated the development of many innovative teams and services that are now well-established and are providing enhanced care for common chronic conditions. A core characteristic of NSF implementation—

Figure 5.3
The Role of Community Matrons

The role of a community matron

They:

Work collaboratively with all professionals, carers and relatives to understand all aspects of the patient's physical, emotional and social situation.

Develop a personalized carre plan with the patient, carers, relatives and health and social care professionals, based on a full assessment of medical, nursing and care needs. The plan includes preventative measures and anticipates any future needs the patient may have.

Keep in touch with the patient and monitor their condition regularly. This may be done by home visits or by telephone contact.

Initiate action if required, such as ordering tests or prescribing.

Update the patient's medical records, including medicines review, and inform other professionals about changes in condition.

Liaise with other local agencies such as social services and the voluntary and community sectors, to mobilize resources as they are needed.

Teach carers and relatives to recognize subtle changes in the patient's condition that could lead to an acute deterioration in their health, and to call for help.

Secure additional support as needed, for example, from home care, intermediate care or paliative care teams, or geriatricians.

Maintain contact with the patient if s/he is admitted to hospital and give the unit treating the patient the information they need to ensure integrated and consistent care.

Note: Reprinted from *Supporting People with Long Term Conditions: An NHS and Social Care Model to Support Local Innovation and Integration* (p. 17), by Department of Health, 2005, London.

and of many of the new services—has been the development of networks and clinical pathways that span community and hospital care. This development has been particularly important in the UK, where GPs have always practiced in the community and specialists have always practiced in hospitals. Links between these two domains have been variable with long delays common if a specialist opinion is needed. The development of specialist "outreach" teams from hospital departments to work closely with GPs, and integrated primary-secondary care pathways, have done a lot to reduce delays and improve the quality of care in relation to common conditions such as asthma, heart failure, and diabetes. Examples of these kinds of developments are given in the Department of Health (2005b) report, *Supporting People with Long Term Conditions*.

Second, the 2004 GP contract introduced micro-incentives (fee-for-service payments) for routine monitoring and enhanced control of seven common long-term conditions: hypertension, coronary heart disease, stroke, diabetes, asthma, COPD, and epilepsy. This new payment system has stimulated GPs to improve their disease registers and develop the systematic, proactive monitoring and treatment arrangements that had been identified in selected high-performing U.S.-managed care organizations.

SELF-MANAGEMENT

The third trench of recent policy has been to develop support for self-management (Department of Health, 2006b). The importance of self-management is recognized at every stage of long-term conditions—from early diagnosis to living with complex illness. To date, policy has focused on the Expert Patient Programme (EPP), a peer learning program for people with long-term conditions. The program provides participants with 10 group sessions led by a trained "expert patient" and covers topics such as coping with pain, managing tiredness, communicating with health professionals, and dealing with difficult emotions. With positive feedback from participants in EPP groups, policy has been to ensure that these courses are available in every Primary Care Trust by 2008 (Department of Health, 2005a). In addition to the EPP, a myriad of other initiatives have developed in an ad hoc way across the country. Patient education groups (e.g., for diabetes or asthma), pharmacy advice clinics, and many other initiatives are underway.

Although the rollout of the EPP is progressing well, many challenges remain in terms of support for self-management. A review of patient views on what is most needed for better self-management indicated that developing the skills of health professionals, and improving information and awareness about local services—for both patients and health professionals—were two key challenges (Corben & Rosen, 2005; Wagner, 1998). These issues are starting to be addressed, but further developments are still needed.

LONG-TERM CONDITIONS POLICY, 2006 ONWARDS

The main policy developments on long-term conditions took place in 2004–2005; however, the issue of improving services and reducing hospital admissions remains high on the government agenda. While not specifically called long-term conditions policy, the subject is prominent in the 2006 White Paper, *Our Health, Our Care, Our Say* (Department of Health, 2006a), which sets out the policy goal of transferring services from hospitals to community settings and defines the ways in which this will be achieved. A key proposal in the White Paper is to establish large-scale "demonstration projects" bringing together health and social care, telemedicine, disease management, and self-management services underpinned by shared health and social care data systems.

These demonstration projects are due to start by the end of 2006 and, importantly, they will be large scale. With the goal of avoiding the prevailing situation where hundreds of small projects are emerging that each reach a few hundred people, the demonstrations will serve populations of 250,000 to 500,000. They will require effective partnerships, not only between health and social care organizations, but also with commercial providers of telemedicine, health informatics services and, perhaps, with voluntary sector organizations and patient groups, too.

CONCLUDING THOUGHTS: WILL RECENT ENGLISH POLICY ACHIEVE ITS GOALS?

On the face of it, the developments described above represent a comprehensive, coherent set of policies aimed at the whole range of people living with long-term conditions. The ingredients of good care are well understood. Policy addresses everything from self-management support for those living full and active lives to intensive service delivery for individuals at highest risk of hospitalization. Some of the infrastructure challenges—the IT and workforce requirements, for example—are also being addressed through other policy initiatives.

However, the context within which all these developments are occurring is problematic. With strong incentives on hospitals to maximize their work (since each admission brings extra money), there is a danger that the broad objective of improving "upstream care" to prevent avoidable admissions will be eclipsed by short-term pressures on hospitals to maximize income. The partnerships that are emerging between generalists and specialists, community and hospital services, and health and social care may be strained by the changing objectives of different participants as the financial incentives bite.

In addition, the use of market forces to drive change in English health services could work either way for long-term conditions. The King's Fund study of chronic disease management in leading U.S.-managed care organizations (Dixon et al., 2004) concluded that competition between providers was a key factor in driving change and innovation. But these providers had problems with continuity of care and with enrollees moving between health plans.

English health care is characterized by continuity of primary care through registration with a single GP, which is a valuable asset for managing long-term conditions. Patient groups representing people with long-term conditions stress the importance of maintaining continuity and argue that patients want high quality, responsive local services rather than the opportunity to choose between providers in a health care market place. The new financial incentives in the English health system risk damaging the emerging relationships between hospitals, GPs, social services, and others aimed at maintaining health and keeping people out of hospital.

This tension between the broad policy objectives of different parts of the health service—planned surgery, long-term conditions, urgent care, prevention—is not unique. But as the population ages and the prevalence of common long-term conditions increases, it will be increasingly important to ensure that the high-level policy jigsaw prioritizes the effective management of long-term conditions. The cost of neglecting them will continue to rise for the foreseeable future.

REFERENCES

Corben, S., & Rosen, R. (2005). *Self-management for long-term conditions: Patients' perspectives on the way ahead.* London: King's Fund. Retrieved October 12, 2006, from http://www.kingsfund.org.uk/resources/publications/selfmanagement.html

Department of Health. (1999a). *National service framework for mental health.* London: Author.

Department of Health. (1999b). *Saving lives: Our healthier nation.* London: Author.

Department of Health. (2000). *National service framework for coronary heart disease.* London: Author.

Department of Health. (2001). *National service framework for older people.* London: Author.

Department of Health. (2002). *National service framework for diabetes.* London: Author.

Department of Health. (2004a). *National service framework for children, young people and maternity services.* London: Author.

Department of Health. (2004b). *The NHS Plan and the new NHS: Providing a patient-centred service.* Retrieved October 12, 2006, from http://www.dh.gov.uk/assetRoot/04/09/25/37/04092537.pdf

Department of Health. (2005a). *Stepping stones to success.* Retrieved October 12, 2006, from http://www.expertpatients.nhs.uk/quality-SteppingStones.shtml

Department of Health. (2005b). *Supporting people with long term conditions: An NHS and social care model to support local innovation and integration.* London: Author.

Department of Health. (2006a). *Our health, our care, our say: A new direction for community services.* London: King's Fund.

Department of Health. (2006b). *Supporting people with long term conditions to self care: A guide to developing local strategies and good practice.* London: Author.

Dixon, J., Lewis, R., Rosen, R., Grey, D., & Finlayson, B. (2004). *Managing chronic disease: What can we learn from the US experience?* Retrieved October 12, 2006, from http://www.kingsfund.org.uk/resources/publications/managing_chronic.html

Feachem, R., Sekhri, N., & White, K. (2002). Getting more for their dollar: A comparison of the NHS with California's Kaiser Permanente. *British Medical Journal, 324,* 135-143.

Lewis, R. (2005). NHS foundation trusts. *British Medical Journal, 331,* 59-60.

Royal College of General Practitioners. (1981). *Health & prevention in primary care. Report of a working party appointed by the Council of the Royal College of General Practitioners.* London: Author.

17 Million Reasons: Unlocking the potential of people with long-term conditions. (2005). Retrieved January 26, 2007, from http://www.17millionreasons.co.uk/

Wagner, E. (1998). Chronic disease management: What will it take to improve care for chronic illness? *Effective Clinical Practice, 1,* 2-4. Retrieved October 12, 2006, from http://www.improvingchroniccare.org/change/model/components.html

CANADIAN INITIATIVES IN CHRONIC DISEASE MANAGEMENT

6. AN OUNCE OF PREVENTION: INTEGRATING CLINICAL PREVENTION INTO FAMILY PRACTICE IN BRITISH COLUMBIA

Shannon Turner

MESH HEADINGS
British Columbia
Chronic disease
Disease management
Family practice
Primary health care
Primary prevention

BACKGROUND

Chronic disease, along with its associated costs, suffering, and premature deaths, is a massive social and financial burden in Canada. The province of British Columbia has recognized the need to address this growing problem and has developed a chronic disease strategy that focuses on both management and prevention. Yet, we find ourselves facing a prevention paradox.

There is clear evidence that prevention activities delivered in primary care reduce the onset of chronic disease. Evidence also shows that preventive interventions are particularly effective when delivered as a multifaceted program tailored to individual primary care practices. Patients expect their family physician to advise them on prevention and healthy lifestyles. Yet, despite medical evidence and public expectations, prevention programs are not being widely delivered in British Columbia.

There is a pressing need to resolve this paradox and enable the primary care system to play a material role in preventing chronic disease. To do this, we must identify and remove barriers at both the clinical and the system level. And this, of course, is where our work begins.

Changing physicians' and patients' long-held patterns of behaviour and clinical working environments is complex and difficult. The task of putting evidence-based preventive care guidelines into practice is especially challenging because of educational, attitudinal, and organizational barriers. Family physicians lack time and resources to carry out and coordinate recommended interventions and many are skeptical about the effectiveness of the recommended preventive services and manoeuvres. Medical Services Commission policies with regard to prevention are under review. Patients also face time, financial, and social restraints. They often fail to see the importance of prevention and have difficulty taking on the responsibility of medical self-management without an easy-to-navigate system of primary support services. Income, education, self-efficacy, and other social determinants of health are key factors that affect patient prevention activities. A social safety net and an efficient, well-organized operating environment are crucial to chronic disease prevention being effective.

Health care managers are increasingly aware of the barriers to prevention, especially the linkage between funding mechanisms and prevention activity. The federal and provincial governments have already taken significant steps toward removing disincentives and enhancing chronic disease prevention. In 2000, the federal government initiated the Primary Health Care Transition Fund (PHCTF) to finance sustainable initiatives that equip and enable the primary health care system to prevent chronic disease. Following on a United States program, Improving Chronic Illness Care (Improving Chronic Illness Care, 2006), British Columbia has developed an Expanded Chronic Care Model that includes health promotion and disease prevention (Barr et al., 2003). The provincial Ministry of Health allocated PCHTF funding and developed a Prevention Flow Sheet as part of the computerized Toolkit for chronic disease management. Health care managers now need substantiated information about current levels of prevention activity, the deterrents to such activity, and solutions.

If British Columbia intends to employ an evidence-based prevention strategy to address the growing burden of chronic disease, and if that strategy depends on the active participation of primary care providers, then those providers must have ready access to a tailored mix of supports at the system and clinical level. The 18-month pilot project presented in this chapter illustrates one approach to prevention.

THE PRIMARY CARE PREVENTION SUPPORT PROGRAM

British Columbia's Primary Care Prevention Support Program (PCPSP) was the product of a powerful interdisciplinary and multijurisdictional partnership. It was federally funded by the PHCTF, which in British Columbia was known as the Primary Care Renewal Health Transition Fund, and administered as the Prevention Support Program. A joint project of the provincial Ministry of Health, Population Health and Wellness, and Primary Care and Chronic Disease Management Divisions, the program was implemented from October 2004 to March 2006 by the British Columbia health authorities in partnership with a core group of primary health care providers.

The Prevention Support Program was intended as a step toward building a health improvement system for British Columbia. The program was designed to promote population health and prevent chronic disease by linking resources within and beyond the health care system. Much more than a screening mechanism, it linked detection with effective treatment and management to integrate chronic disease prevention in primary health care with chronic disease management. The purpose of the Prevention Support Program was to create a system that does not depend solely on additional sustained funding, but on better integration of existing resources.

MACRO-LEVEL ELEMENTS

With high-level public policy focused on primary health care renewal, and the current emphasis on prevention, the Prevention Support Program reaped the advantages of good timing and a supportive policy environment. The pilot program was funded by Health Canada's PHCTF initiative, which is designed to facilitate systemic, long-term renewal by supporting Canada's provinces and territories in their efforts to improve delivery of primary health care services. A major strategy of British Columbia's grant portion was to improve health outcomes, with a focus on Chronic Disease Management (CDM). A strategic partnership was established between the Ministry of Health and health authorities. The ministry establishes policy and standards; the health authorities plan, implement, and deliver services in their regions. The Prevention Support Program was developed as part of the province's health care renewal activities.

British Columbia has developed a chronic disease strategy with two main elements: *manage* diseases more efficiently and effectively, and *prevent* their development in the future. The dual approaches of chronic disease management and prevention were integrated into the Expanded Chronic Care Model—a British Columbia version of the Chronic Care Model that had been developed in the United States—resulting in an effective framework for reducing the growth and impact of chronic disease. The Expanded Chronic Care Model was used as the overall guiding framework for the Prevention Support Program. It calls for health care to be reengineered to create an environment in which efforts to prevent and manage chronic disease are systematically supported, encouraged, and rewarded. The model also values the role of community resources in addressing barriers to achieving prevention goals, especially social-environmental factors that determine long-term success. In keeping with the model's guiding principles, the Prevention Support Program included the following elements: an agreed-upon set of relevant goals and objectives, visible and tangible top leadership support for prevention goals at the health authority, and system-level policy initiatives that promote and enable clinical preventive services.

The Prevention Support Program was the result of a coordinated effort among some of Canada's best thinkers, researchers, managers, policy makers, and clinical leaders in primary care and chronic disease prevention. Three inter-cooperative bodies made up the program leadership profile: the Program Steering Committee, an Expert Advisory Group, and the Provincial Coordinator.

The Program Steering Committee included representatives from British Columbia's five health authorities, the Ministry of Health, and family practice physicians. By examining existing programs, the steering committee defined strategies most suitable for putting prevention into practice, and established the program's overall direction. The committee then planned the infrastructure for the prevention collaborative and developed and tested prevention flow charts, in partnership with collaborative physicians, to assist in implementing the program. Finally, the steering committee was responsible for resolving operational issues that crossed over health authority jurisdictions, and for monitoring the program's progress and performance.

The Expert Advisory Group included national leaders and key stakeholders in primary care and clinical prevention research. Its advisory role focused on prevention priorities, increasing uptake of effective interventions, and evaluation criteria. The group participated in a province-wide collaborative session where it listened to provincial opportunities and challenges, and responded by recommending policy and program improvements. Furthermore, the Expert Advisory Group worked to remove barriers against implementing prevention by identifying national influences on systemic change.

The provincial coordinator was responsible for leading project implementation by overseeing and supporting program design and delivery across the province. The coordinator acted as liaison with the Expert Advisory Group and facilitated the Provincial Steering Committee. The work of the coordinator involved establishing a training program and network for provincial facilitators, communicating PCPSP protocols to undertake baseline audits and flow sheet utilization, ensuring independent evaluation, conducting site visits, leading collaborative meetings, communicating clinical evidence and policy challenges to constituents, and managing data extracts and analysis for program surveillance. Along with the Expert Advisory Group, the provincial coordinator identified systemic change to remove barriers to implementing prevention. Overall, the coordinator performed a key role as "champion" for the project by seeking new collaborative opportunities and spreading the news.

Work done at this level resulted in the following strategic decisions:

- The Prevention Support Program was built onto the successful CDM project—the Expanded Chronic Care Model—and used the CDM Toolkit to facilitate implementation in the available time frame.
- Eleven category "A/B" evidence-based prevention manoeuvres were selected from the Canadian Taskforce on Preventive Services Guide to be applied in clinical settings.
- The cohort was limited to patients aged 50 to 70 as a manageable target, considering workload and timeline for the Prevention Support Program.
- Based on the project budget, timelines, and constraints clinicians were facing, the PCPSP focused on opportunistic prevention.

MESO-LEVEL ELEMENTS

The Prevention Support Program was implemented through the health authorities. Four of the five health authorities chose to participate based on their interest and capacity. The Fraser Health Authority did not participate because its own prevention initiative—the implementation of an electronic health record—was already underway. The Fraser Health Authority gave its funding allotment back to the PCPSP project to be used by other health authorities; however, it maintained representation on the Steering Committee. Uptake of the Prevention Support Program reflected its perceived value. Conceptually, it offered health authorities an excellent opportunity to develop partnerships with and among primary health care providers, provided them with a better idea of their current levels of prevention, and pointed to opportunities for improvement.

It was up to individual health authorities to develop a plan that identified their own approach to prevention support, focusing on primary care providers and organizations deemed most suitable in their own area. Incentives unique to each health authority were developed to compensate participating physicians for their project-related activities, such as compiling baseline data. Participating health authorities were funded for additional staff, travel, and training. The Vancouver Island Health Authority played a leading role in project implementation and was additionally funded for a provincial project coordinator and support staff.

Staff included 11 experienced and knowledgeable nurse prevention facilitators who offered practical assistance and support to team members and facilitated the team's commitment to health promotion. A proven set of workshops and educational materials were used to train the facilitators, consultants, and auditors to deliver the Prevention Support Program. Training was provided by the University of Ottawa Institute of Population Health team of Lemelin, Hogg and Baskerville, who had conducted an Ontario study that engaged a tailored, multifaceted approach to changing family physician practice patterns and improving preventive care (2001). The facilitation model created by the Ontario team provided an operational framework for the Prevention Support Program. Curriculum was adapted to the British Columbia context by the provincial coordinator, Shannon Turner, in partnership with Eileen Vilis of the University of Ottawa Institute of Population Health.

MICRO-LEVEL ELEMENTS

At the provider level, the trained prevention facilitators secured participation commitments from practices throughout British Columbia. Forty physicians, in four health authorities, participated in the program. Ancillary participants included dietitians, medical office assistants, CDM nurses, and nurse practitioners. A total of 6,000 patients, aged 50 to 70, were included in the study. The practices reviewed 200 random charts of 2004 data, within the cohort of patients aged 50 to 70, to establish a baseline reference. Support for this intervention included the baseline flow sheet and assistance from a prevention facilitator. The chart audit provided a snapshot of existing levels of prevention activities for each practice.

At the clinical level, it was crucial to provide participating practices with a system of supports to assist in making the necessary changes to plan and deliver prevention services. The nurse prevention facilitators helped to plan and implement a tailored Prevention Support Program for each practice, according to the needs and capacities of individual practitioners and practice environments. This included implementing 11 selected prevention manoeuvres. Each facilitator assumed an ongoing role as a resource and liaison between the various operational elements of the program, such as data recording, monitoring, and feedback. Participating health care workers were provided with education and training, including workshops on evidence-based prevention by the University of Ottawa team.

Feedback loops were established, including routine reports on prevention performance for individual practices and for the overall program. Reminder systems and tools were introduced and reviewed, including preventive care flow sheets, the CDM Toolkit, chart stamps and stickers, and recall initiatives. As well, patient education materials from credible sources were provided and updated. Due to the short time-frame of the initiative, recall was not a major focus of the program. However, several clinicians, motivated by the report capability of the CDM Toolkit, made significant improvements in intervention-specific recall systems.

A clinical information system was introduced to provide timely information and reminders about individual patients, and populations of patients, with chronic disease issues. The information system supported participating practices by identifying individuals and populations at risk, summarizing the status of preventive services on a patient's chart, and prompting planned preventive care. Practices were provided with routine feedback on performance in meeting their prevention goals. Physicians also had access to a secure website with electronic flow sheets and patient treatment schedules. A listserv was established to enable participating physicians to communicate with each other, share observations, and comment on the efficiencies of the new system.

Processes to enhance patient self-management formed an integral part of the program. Physicians were supported in helping their patients to recognize their need for preventive services and to take action to obtain them. Patients were included in collaborative efforts to set goals and identify personal barriers to prevention. Patients were offered self-help materials, referrals to appropriate community-based agencies, and follow-up support.

OUTCOMES

Primary care providers who participated in the Prevention Support Program report that they are now more aware of prevention in their overall practice, not only within the 50-to-70-age-group cohort. They also report a continuing increase in the use of preventive manoeuvres in their practice and, in particular, implementing manoeuvres starting at the point of highest risk for the patient. Overall, participants in this project are finding that implementing prevention is improving physician-patient relationships.

Data extracted from the provincial registry, for selected interventions for appropriate populations, show a range of 10% to 30% increase in manoeuvres over the course of the pilot project in comparison to baseline. Individual practitioners may have reported even more significant increases as a result of particular quality improvement activities. This is consistent with the findings of Lemelin, Hogg, and Baskerville (2001), who demonstrated a 20% increase in appropriate interventions, compared with the control group, over an 18-month period. In a process evaluation of the same project, they found that the key interventions were audit and feedback on prevention performance, consensus on a prevention plan, and reminder systems.

LESSONS LEARNED

Having completed our 18-month odyssey of planning, implementing, and evaluating our Prevention Support Program, we have identified a number of elements that worked particularly well in moving the project forward.

We began with strong leadership from the Program Steering Committee and the British Columbia Ministry of Health. In addition, the presence of an Expert Advisory Group allowed timely access to the best and most current information on prevention implementation and policy. The program leadership bodies formed a powerful partnership with unique jurisdictional crossover and strategic placement of the provincial coordinator, a key resource, within one of the participating health authorities. Consequently, mentoring, trust, and information sharing were established early in the planning stages and resulted in highly productive collaborative discussions.

Organizational tools, such as the PCPSP logic model and evaluation framework, clearly set out the program goals, objectives, and guiding principles so that all participating individuals, groups, and organizations worked according to the same guidelines. Implementation tools, such as the prevention flow sheets and electronic CDM Toolkit, increased the efficiency and consistency of data collection.

A key element to this effort is understanding the important role of the multidisciplinary primary care team. We worked with a committed team of primary care coordinators and facilitators. Physician investment of time was critical, as was nursing and dietitian support, and building the capacity of medical office assistants—the front lines of clinical care—to partner in clinical prevention.

We also encountered a number of challenges that impeded the progress of the program. Time and money forced an opportunistic focus on prevention, rather than the planned prevention strategy preferred by clinicians. Because fee-for-service physicians, salaried physicians, and nurse practitioners operate in different environments, the implementation model had to be adaptive in order to support a diverse range of service delivery models. The 18-month time frame for implementation and assessment was very short and resulted in the lack of an effective recall system. There were also a number of challenges relating to privacy legislation and the data extraction process from the Ministry of Health. In addition, the effectiveness of the CDM Toolkit, a key implementation tool, was compromised by delays in reports and updates, and limited support. However, physicians and medical office assistants managed to work effectively with the program in spite of this limitation. Focused meetings were required to address these barriers and attend to program deliverables.

RECOMMENDATIONS

For prevention-based health care to become a reality, a number of systemic changes must take place. The PCPSP pilot program has resulted in a number of primary recommendations:

- Establish a prevention-friendly policy environment.
- Establish incentives through funding models that support clinical prevention of chronic disease.
- Conduct a cost-benefit analysis to determine the true cost of prevention, considering return on investment.
- Improve information management and technology supports such as electronic medical records and the CDM Toolkit .
- Address privacy impact assessment and legislation regarding clinical registries.
- Expedite the data extraction process from the Ministry of Health.
- Further develop the role of the Expert Advisory Group.
- Advocate for the facilitation model and physician collaboratives as a successful implementation strategy.
- Support clinicians in delivering planned prevention versus opportunistic prevention.
- Continue to partner with CDM initiatives because chronic disease management is a priority in family practice.

The PCPSP pilot project demonstrated that a multi-pronged approach that combines an interdisciplinary team, decision support instruments, facilitation, and medical leadership can deliver dramatic results in compressed time frames. It is possible to work effectively across jurisdictions in complex service delivery environments when partners are committed, evidence is utilized, and leadership is shared at every level of governance. Early results indicate that it is time to take the next step and institute prevention as a primary focus for clinical care in Canada.

ACKNOWLEDGEMENTS

This project could not have been accomplished without the generous support of these key people. Valerie Tregillus and Howard Platt, BC Ministry of Health, helped make room for clinical prevention in the primary care agenda. Andy Hazelwood and Trevor Hancock spearheaded the proposal for this initiative. Dr. Richard Stanwick, Chief Medical Health Officer, and Sylvia Robinson, Director of Public Health for Vancouver Island Health Authority (VIHA), gave the Prevention Support Program a home. Dr. Richard Nuttall, an early advocate for prevention, brought his experience in community medicine and as a medical health officer to this work in his family practice and served as VIHA's clinical lead. The facilitation coordinators blazed the trail, taking the evidence forward to family doctors and creating supportive environments for this transition. Our Expert Advisory Group—Dr. Frederic Bass, Dr. Daniel MacCarthy, Dr. John Freightner, Dr. Vivian Ramsden, Dr. William Hogg, Dr. John Miller, and Dr. Bob Wollard—provided consultative and policy leadership. Dr. Gregory Taylor, Public Health Agency of Canada, made the trek westward to our provincial congress to inspire and inform our community partners. The Provincial Steering Committee delivered sound and pragmatic leadership throughout this process.

I owe many thanks to the physicians who gave their time to test and improve the prevention flow sheet: to Dr. Trevor Corneil, Dr. Richard Crow, and Dr. Art Macgregor who took time from exceptionally busy lives to come and speak to our coordinators as they prepared to launch this initiative; and to Eileen Vilis, Jackie Schultz, and Dr. William Hogg, Institute of Population Health, University of Ottawa, who provided training and expertise on putting prevention into practice. I extend a special thank you to Dr. Art Macgregor who, as senior medical lead of VIHA's Chronic Disease Management Initiative, cajoled, challenged, improved, and fought for the best prevention program we could build. All of you have shaped a useful beginning.

REFERENCES

Barr, V., Robinson, S., Marin-Link, B., Underhill, L., Dotts, A., Ravensdale, D., & Salivaras, S. (2003). The Expanded Chronic Care Model: An integration of concepts and strategies from population health promotion and the Chronic Care Model. *Hospital Quarterly, 7*(1), 73-82.

Improving Chronic Illness Care. (2006). Retrieved May 23, 2006, from http://www.improvingchroniccare.org/about/index1.html

Lemelin, J., Hogg, W., & Baskerville, N. (2001). Evidence to action: A tailored multifaceted approach to changing family physician practice patterns and improving preventive care. *Canadian Medical Association Journal, 164*(6), 757-763.

7. THE SASKATCHEWAN CHRONIC DISEASE MANAGEMENT COLLABORATIVE

Ben Chan, on behalf of the Health Quality Council Chronic Disease Management Collaborative Team

MESH HEADINGS
Chronic disease
Coronary arteriosclerosis
Diabetes mellitus
Disease management
Medical records systems, computerized
Physician incentive plans
Quality assurance, health care
Saskatchewan

BACKGROUND

Chronic disease management is an area ripe for quality improvement. Major chronic diseases account for a large share of the burden of illness. In Canada, the prevalence of diabetes among those aged 20 and over was 4.4% in 1999–2000 (Centre for Chronic Disease Prevention and Control, 2002); in Saskatchewan, diabetes prevalence has increased by 41% from 1996–97 to 2000–01 (Osei & Hawkey, 2003). Cardiovascular disease is the leading cause of mortality in Canada (Heart and Stroke Foundation, 2003) and accounts for $18 billion in direct and indirect costs (Strategic Policy Directorate, 2002). Many studies identify deficiencies in care. In the United States, only 56% of recommended best practices for chronic conditions in primary care settings are routinely delivered (McGlynn et al., 2003). In Saskatchewan, reports from the Health Quality Council highlight suboptimal use of evidence-based medications following an acute myocardial infarction (Chan et al., 2004). Furthermore, less than half of diabetes patients achieve optimal management of lipid levels and long-term glucose control, as measured by A1C levels (Chan, Klomp, Cascagnette, & Brossart, 2006).

A naive view of why chronic disease management is suboptimal is that physicians do not keep up to date with practice guidelines. The reality is far more complex. Most care systems are provider-centric and do not support team-based care. This imposes barriers to communication and provision of care by the most appropriate provider at the right time. Many physicians find that patient adherence to recommendations is a challenge, and feel frustrated by the limited amount of time to address complex disease management issues. From the patient's perspective, the way in which information is presented may affect adherence. Simply being told repeatedly what to do does not make the patient feel truly engaged in important decisions regarding their care.

Wagner's Chronic Care Model (see chapter 1) contains potent ideas for improving care. It emphasizes self-management support, decision support tools, delivery system design, clinical information systems, and effective partnerships with community resources. Patient self-management involves helping the patient set individualized goals, identify barriers to change, and develop individualized strategies to address these barriers. Decision support tools provide practitioners with reminders or information as needed on what are the most appropriate practices in a given situation. Delivery system design means optimally using the members of the team and designing the flow of care around the patient's needs, not the provider's convenience. Clinical information systems can help care providers track all patients with chronic disease, and can inform the provider as to what the current quality of care is across different indicators, whether or not quality is improving over time, and which subpopulations need more urgent or targeted attention. Coordination of efforts across community partners and providers reduces duplication of services and allows patients to access the right person at the right time for the right information, intervention, and support.

Primary care practices that successfully implement the ideas for improvement embedded in Wagner's model have rich knowledge of the "how" of implementation. If, for example, they implement effective patient self-management strategies, they can credibly sell the concept to others. If they improve their team functioning, they may have insight into how they overcame typical team conflicts or engaged different health professionals. Such experiential information is not typically taught in traditional continuing professional education courses, which tend to focus only on "what" is the best practice to be applied. Indeed, if quality improvement activities take place in one site in isolation from other sites, then there is no way of sharing such information and the opportunity to spread change is lost.

Quality improvement advocates have recognized the need for formal structures to spread these experiences of implementing best practices. A *collaborative* (also known as Learning Collaborative) is a carefully designed quality improvement method aimed at rapidly spreading best practices across multiple teams interested in a common topic. This method was developed by the Institute for Healthcare Improvement in the United States in 1995 (Institute for Healthcare Improvement, 2003). The standard collaborative model brings quality improvement teams with a common aim to four learning workshops within 6 to 15 months to teach them basic quality improvement skills and change concepts that they can apply in their local settings. Teams implement different ideas for change and share their experiences at subsequent workshops.

Collaboratives have generated important quality improvements in many areas, particularly chronic disease management. Collaboratives in congestive heart failure have been shown to improve drug management (Asch et al., 2005), and, in an Australian example, to reduce readmissions from 7.2% to 2.4% (Scott et al., 2004). Two diabetes collaboratives in Washington State involving 47 teams demonstrated improvements in blood sugar testing and control, blood pressure control, lipid testing and control, use of foot exams, dilated eye exams, and self-management goals (Daniel et al., 2004). Another diabetes collaborative in Washington State showed similar results, with the greatest gains in community health centres with the fewest resources servicing the most challenging patients (Wagner et al., 2001).

PROGRAM DESCRIPTION

The Saskatchewan Chronic Disease Management Collaborative was formally launched in November 2005. It aims to improve diabetes, coronary artery disease, and clinical office design (also known as advanced access or improved access). The decision to tackle three areas simultaneously was made because both diabetes and coronary artery disease are very common conditions, and many best practices for managing these diseases are similar (e.g., tight blood pressure and lipid control). Furthermore, clinical office redesign provides tools to assist practices in reducing wait times—a significant issue in providing effective chronic care—and also improves processes to better meet the needs of all patients.

The aims of the Saskatchewan Collaborative (Table 7.1) were set by a reference panel consisting of local and international experts. This panel met prior to the start of the initial learning workshop. For selected measures, the goal was that three-quarters of patients would meet their targets for optimal management. As noted previously, in many instances only half of the patients received optimal care. Therefore, these aims were intended to cut by 50% the instances of suboptimal care.

This initiative is being led and funded by Saskatchewan's Health Quality Council (HQC), in partnership with all 13 health regions, several First Nations and Métis organizations, and the Saskatchewan Department of Health. The HQC also received training and support on how to run collaboratives from the United Kingdom's National Primary Care Development Team (now called the Improvement Foundation), which has had extensive experience in implementing such initiatives. Like other collaboratives, there are four learning workshops within a year, at which participants engage in plenary sessions and small group discussions on quality improvement tools and change ideas. Participants also share their learnings with each other using storyboard presentations (see Figure 7.1). The Saskatchewan Collaborative is being run in two waves, each commencing one year apart, with different participants in each wave.

Table 7.1
Aims of the Saskatchewan Chronic Disease Management Collaborative

Diabetes
- 75% will have A1C ≤ 7%
- 75% will have BP ≤ 130/80
- 75% will have TC/HDL ratio < 4.0

Coronary artery disease
- 75% will have anti-platelet therapy
- 75% will have BP ≤ 140/90 or ≤ 130/80
- 75% will have TC/HDL ratio < 4.0

Improved access
- 80% will be seen on their day of choice

Note: The A1C test measures long-term blood sugar control. BP = blood pressure. TC = total cholesterol. HDL = high-density lipoprotein cholesterol.

Figure 7.1
Storyboard from the Saskatchewan Chronic Disease Management Collaborative

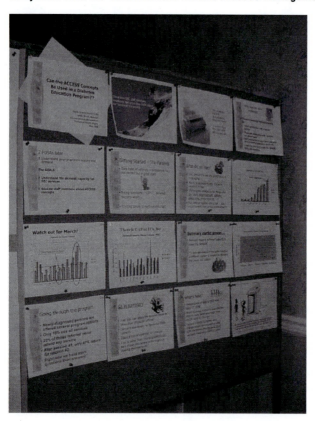

Participants learn about the Model for Improvement, which ensures that all quality improvement teams answer three key questions: What are we trying to accomplish? How will we know if a change is an improvement? And, what changes can we make that will result in improvement? The model also promotes frequent small tests of change, or Plan-Do-Study-Act (PDSA) cycles (Langley, Nolan, Nolan, Norman, & Provost, 1996). Quality improvement teams are encouraged to identify different activities or changes to processes of care that could improve quality. Teams test the ideas on a very small scale, monitor the results, then modify and retest, repeating the PDSA cycle multiple times. Eventually, teams identify a method of implementing a best practice that works best in their local environment. In between learning workshops, teams engage in action periods where they apply the Model for Improvement and PDSA cycles to test different change ideas in their practices, and then share their learnings with their peers at the next learning workshop.

PARTICIPANTS IN THE COLLABORATIVE AND QUALITY IMPROVEMENT (QI) TEAMS

Participants in the Saskatchewan Chronic Disease Management Collaborative include the broadest possible spectrum of providers involved in the delivery of services for diabetes and coronary artery disease. Within the existing system, the level of integration of services among providers working in the same geographic location is less than optimal. The collaborative is attempting to build linkages between different provider groups and to significantly enhance teamwork.

Within the Saskatchewan Collaborative, QI teams exist at two levels. First, family physician practices need to function better as a team to implement changes within their own practices, such as the introduction of flow sheets and data entry. Participants in these activities include family physicians, their office staff, and other health providers in their workplace.

Secondly, regional improvement teams were created within each health region. Members of these teams include representatives from participating family physician practices, health region staff involved in the delivery of chronic disease care such as nurses, diabetes educators, nutritionists, and pharmacists, as well as First Nations and Métis health personnel and patients. These teams are exploring opportunities to increase the proportion of patients attaining optimal management through better patient flow, communication, and coordination of care.

Each health region was asked to recruit at least one non-fee-for-service practice (known in Saskatchewan as a primary health care site), but no more than 50% of practices could be these primary health care sites. Recruitment was open to solo and group practices as well as remote sites served primarily by nurse practitioners, in order to promote sharing and innovation across multiple practice models. Each practice sent one representative physician (typically the same individual) to each learning workshop, along with an office manager or medical office assistant. Such office staff were considered crucial partners in redesigning office flow to improve both access and clinical care for chronic disease patients. For primary health care sites, an additional member of the team, such as a nurse practitioner, also attended the workshops. Three representatives of each regional improvement team who were not part of a practice attended the learning workshops as well.

SUPPORT FOR QI TEAMS

Providing topic expertise, mentorship, and support to participants is an important determinant of success. The Saskatchewan Chronic Disease Management Collaborative has made four physicians available, one to act as a clinical lead in each of the three topic areas and a fourth to act as overall clinical chair.[1] These individuals are available throughout the collaborative process to give general advice to participants. The HQC also funded and hired collaborative facilitators in each health region to act as QI advisors to the regional improvement teams and individual physician practices. The collaborative facilitators and regional improvement teams are supported and mentored by HQC staff. On average, there is one full-time equivalent staff person to provide support for every four participating practice teams. For each wave of the Saskatchewan Collaborative, participants will have access to these advisory services for at least several months after the end of the last learning workshop.

TOOLS FOR IMPROVEMENT

The HQC also provided participants with a 131-page handbook (Health Quality Council, 2005) containing information about the Saskatchewan Collaborative, the Model for Improvement, and specific change concepts and ideas. Many of these ideas were identified from the best practices literature and were organized by the different components of an expanded version of Wagner's Chronic Care Model. The manual also includes examples of PDSA cycles conducted in practice sites in the United Kingdom, British Columbia, and Saskatchewan (see Figure 7.2).

Wagner's Chronic Care Model emphasizes the importance of clinical information systems. One of the cornerstones of the Saskatchewan Collaborative was the development and support of a web-based patient registry, known as the Chronic Disease Management (CDM) Toolkit. This software application was adapted from one used in British Columbia (see chapter 3) in such a way that the CDM Toolkit could in the future connect with other parts of the provincial information technology infrastructure when they are built. This will allow, for example, lab data to automatically flow to the CDM Toolkit when the lab database becomes available. Responsibilities for developing and funding the Toolkit were shared between the HQC and the Saskatchewan Department of Health.

The first step in populating the web-based registry was to identify patients with diabetes and coronary artery disease. Participating physicians signed a "Request for Probabilistic List" letter allowing the Saskatchewan Department of Health to generate, based on the physician billing number, a list of those

Figure 7.2
Example of Plan-Do-Study-Act (PDSA) Cycle

PDSA Cycle—Cycle 1	
PLAN *What is the object of this improvement cycle? Who is involved? What? When? Where? Why? What do we predict will happen? What additional information will we need to take action?*	Purpose of the cycle: To choose a patient self-management goal sheet for tracking and inclusion into patient chart. Our intent is to test two different patient self-management goal sheets to determine which one is the most functional. One of these forms is a check-off form with 10 top goals listed. The other requires the patient to choose and write down their own goals. We are going to test these on two patients each at their next visit. We expect we will be able to determine which form our clinical champion, nurse and patients prefer to use.
DO *Was the test carried out as planned? What did we observe that was not part of the plan?*	We downloaded the two forms from the web site: www.A1cnow.net. We employed the forms on the first two diabetic patients that we saw. We had them fill out both forms and then asked them which they preferred. Both patients chose the same form.
STUDY *How did or didn't the results agree with the predictions we made earlier? What new knowledge was gained through this cycle?*	Both patients selected the form that our clinical champion and nurse preferred. Our initial feeling was that patients would prefer a form that did not require them to write a lot of information down. We felt they would prefer a form that would allow them to simply check off their goals. We found that they actually preferred a combination of the two forms. They wanted a form that would allow them to check off their goals but also to write down anything not listed that they felt was important.
ACT *Now what? Do we abandon? adjust? adopt? Are there forces in our organization that will help or hinder these changes? Objective of next cycle?*	We will be changing the form to allow space for those patients who do want to write in a goal to be able to do so. We will be using the form with the next 5 diabetic patients from our registry.

Note: Reprinted from the *Saskatchewan Chronic Disease Management Handbook*, by the Health Quality Council, 2005, Saskatoon, SK: Author.

patients in their care who likely had diabetes and/or coronary artery disease. The Department then ran an algorithm designed by the HQC for identifying patients with diabetes or coronary artery disease based on physician billing, drug prescribing, and hospitalization data. The algorithm erred on being more sensitive than specific. This list of patients was then uploaded into the physician's account within the CDM Toolkit. Physicians then reviewed the charts of these patients to see if they truly had diabetes or coronary artery disease, and revised their patient list accordingly.

Following the orientation learning workshop, office staff entered clinical flow-sheet data on each patient for the baseline period, which extended from the current time to the previous 12 to 24 months. Examples of information recorded include A1C, blood pressure, cholesterol levels, weight, smoking status, and use of recommended medications (see Figure 7.3). Baseline results were presented to participating practices in the subsequent learning workshop. Physician practices continually added new information with subsequent patient visits and lab tests. Physicians, as trustees of the patient record, also authorized access to the CDM Toolkit to other care providers, such as dietitians, so that they too could enter new clinical information, thereby improving communication and coordination of care.

The CDM Toolkit provided wave 1 practices with run charts for key measures, bar charts comparing anonymously their results with other practices, and recall reports identifying patients who were overdue for selected procedures and interventions. For wave 2, practices using selected electronic medical record systems will be able to exchange clinical data with the CDM Toolkit. A major enhancement to British Columbia's application was the creation of a PDSA catalogue—an electronic repository of all practice improvements tried by practices and regional improvement teams participating in the Saskatchewan Collaborative.

Figure 7.3
Snapshot of the Diabetes Flow Sheet Used in Web-Based Patient Registry

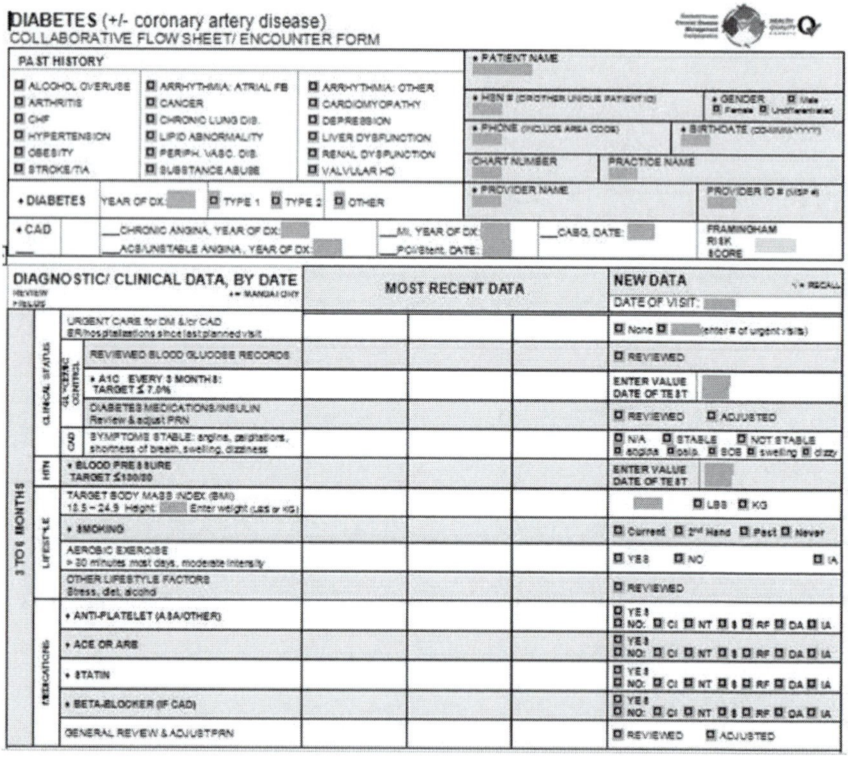

PHYSICIAN RECRUITMENT EFFORTS

For each health region, the aim was to recruit 20% of all physician practices in the first wave. This strategy of aggressive recruitment is similar to that used by the Improvement Foundation in the United Kingdom. According to Rogers' (1995) diffusion of innovation theory, when a large enough group of early adopters accepts a change, there reaches a tipping point where the change begins to spread more rapidly to other members of the system. The 20% threshold represents the "innovators," "early adopters," and some of the "early majority" as described by Rogers (1995). By this logic, if the early recruitment captures only a small proportion of the innovators or early adopters, then change initiatives may be stuck in a prolonged period of pilot testing before widespread adoption.

The HQC mounted an aggressive physician recruitment campaign. This included information sessions hosted in multiple local communities throughout the province and information teleconferences for interested physicians. The Saskatchewan Medical Association supported the recruitment by including promotional articles about the CDM Collaborative in its newsletter to all physicians in the province. HQC staff also met with senior leadership teams and CEOs from each of the health regions to secure their support for the initiative. Lastly, wave 1 physicians were asked to encourage colleagues in their own regions to join wave 2 of the Saskatchewan Collaborative.

Physicians were offered a reimbursement package for the expenses related to participating in the collaborative. This package included a lump sum payment intended to subsidize the costs of travel, IT upgrades (e.g., high speed Internet access and up-to-date computers, if not already available), and time away from clinical practice, which would mean loss of income for fee-for-service physicians or the cost of physician backfill. Attendance at learning workshops was a prerequisite for receiving remuneration. Physician practices also received a $5 per patient subsidy for the costs of entering baseline data into the web-based registry.

As an additional incentive, physicians could also obtain MAINPRO-C and MAINPRO-M1 credits from the College of Family Physicians of Canada for participating in the learning workshops. Such credits are necessary for certified family physicians to maintain their certification. Because the learning workshops were accredited learning events, physicians were also eligible for reimbursement from the Saskatchewan Medical Association's continuing medical education fund.

OUTCOMES

The Saskatchewan CDM Collaborative successfully recruited 35 family physician practices—representing 130 physicians and 16% of the family physician workforce in the province—in the first wave. Approximately 7,800 patients with diabetes or coronary artery disease were entered into the patient registry.

At least one physician practice from each of the 13 health regions of the province participated in the collaborative. All but two practices maintained participation for the duration of wave 1. In wave 2, 41 practices were recruited, but a smaller number of new physicians (60) joined. In total, one-quarter of the entire family physician workforce in Saskatchewan signed on to either wave 1 or 2.

Preliminary results from wave 1 are encouraging. For patients with diabetes, in the 9 months after the baseline period there has been a 39% relative increase in microalbumin screening, a 27% increase in ASA prescribing, and a 16% increase in statin prescribing (Figure 7.4). For patients with coronary artery disease, there was an 11% relative increase in statin use and an 11% increase in ASA prescribing (Figure 7.5). Intermediate outcomes in general are harder to impact than process of care measures. However, the collaborative practices still experienced a 9% relative increase in the proportion of diabetes patients meeting their targets for blood pressure control, and a 6% increase for attaining optimal A1C control. It is anticipated that gains will continue to be made over the next year.

Figure 7.4
Run Chart for Quality Indicators for Diabetes Patients in the Saskatchewan Chronic Disease Management Collaborative, 2006

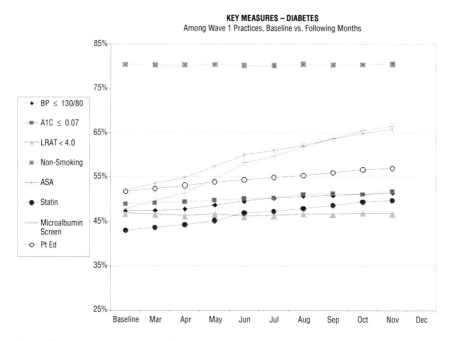

Note: BP = blood pressure. The A1C test measures long-term blood sugar control. LRAT = lipid ratio. ASA = acetylsalicylic acid. PtEd = patient education.

Figure 7.5
Run Chart for Quality Indicators for Coronary Artery Disease Patients in the Saskatchewan Chronic Disease Management Collaborative, 2006

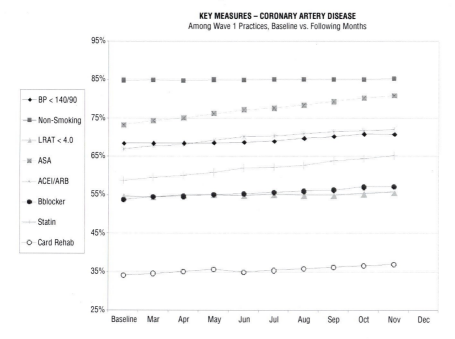

KEY MEASURES – CORONARY ARTERY DISEASE
Among Wave 1 Practices, Baseline vs. Following Months

Note: BP = blood pressure. LRAT = lipid ratio. ASA = acetylsalicylic acid. ACEI/ARB = angiotensin converting enzyme inhibitor or angiotensin II receptor blocker. Bblocker = beta-blocker. Card Rehab = referral to cardiac rehabilitation.

LESSONS LEARNED

THE COLLABORATIVE APPROACH AS A MEANS OF SPREADING PRACTICE

On average, it takes 15 to 20 years for evidence to be adopted into practice (Balas & Boren, 2000). The CDM Collaborative approach shrinks this long time lag, by providing a structured approach to spreading ideas and experiences on how to implement best practices.

TEAM INVOLVEMENT

Local team structures likely contributed to the early successes seen to date. For example, in many regions, physicians are providing community providers access to information in the web-based registry and allowing them to update

information from their encounters. This is one example of increased communication and coordination between different providers.

One of the key team members, in this case, is the medical office assistant or
office manager. These individuals are often left out of decision making, and
they greatly appreciated the opportunity to participate. Indeed, they often became the champions for quality improvement within the office setting and, in
some instances, getting their buy-in was a critical factor in physician
recruitment.

EXTENSIVE TEAM SUPPORT

Quality improvement methods are still new to Saskatchewan. For many participants, the Model for Improvement and PDSA cycles represent a new way
of thinking. Success depends on providing time-intensive support to participants. Following the end of the four learning workshops of wave 1, participants
asked the HQC to consider other means of ensuring ongoing support. Ideas
for how to provide this support are currently under development.

REIMBURSING PHYSICIANS FOR THE COSTS OF PARTICIPATING IN QI INITIATIVES

Participation in QI activities requires time. For fee-for-service physicians, this
means time away from practice and therefore loss of revenue. For alternate
payment physicians, time away may mean costs to hire a locum, or increased
workload stress from having to clear patient backlogs upon their return. Participation in the collaborative means increased staff time for data entry and
participation in QI activities. Ultimately, the physician or non-fee-for-service
clinic may need to pay for increased staff hours. For these reasons, at least
partial reimbursement was essential to securing physician participation.

The HQC was not in a position to reimburse all of the costs of participation, especially costs such as the time needed to participate in QI activities. At
the conclusion of the wave 1 learning workshops, physicians were surveyed
as to what extent the availability of financial compensation influenced their
decision to participate in the Saskatchewan CDM Collaborative. Among
respondents, 36% responded "not at all," 33% responded "moderate," and 30%
replied "a great deal." At the time of press, the Saskatchewan Medical Association had just secured additional funding for chronic disease management,
which may help recruitment efforts in the future.

It should be emphasized that reimbursement for the costs of participating
in QI activities is fundamentally different from pay-for-performance schemes
currently in place in some jurisdictions, such as the United Kingdom, and
selected insurance plans or health maintenance organizations in the United
States. Cost reimbursement simply recognizes the costs of participating. The
payment is not contingent on improvement, which helps avoid any potential
gaming of the system.

SECURING THE SUPPORT OF KEY PHYSICIAN ORGANIZATIONS AND OPINION LEADERS

The support of the Saskatchewan Medical Association in making information about the CDM Collaborative available to its members was an important factor in recruitment. The clinical leads and chair were front-line family physicians, not specialists, who could be considered as peers to the target audience of family physicians. In some regions, other physician champions, such as chiefs of staff, also provided great assistance to recruitment efforts. Wave 1 physicians also helped to recruit wave 2 physicians.

SECURING THE SUPPORT OF HEALTH REGIONS

The vast majority of family physicians are not employees of health regions. However, having the leadership of the health region visibly behind the CDM Collaborative made an important difference in several instances. For example, in one region that overshot its target for recruitment in wave 2, the senior leadership sponsored informal information sharing events such as summer barbecues to encourage strong participation at team meetings, and personally encouraged new physicians to join in the second wave.

SUMMARY

Spreading best practices for chronic disease management requires highly co-ordinated, intensive activities. Traditional passive approaches involving dissemination of guidelines or lectures do not adequately teach the "how" of improvement. Collaboratives provide a formal process for teaching the how of improvement. Ambitious enrolment targets, "stretch goals" for improvement, and intensive support for spread activities are a powerful combination to shrink the long gap in adoption of best evidence.

ACKNOWLEDGEMENTS—THE HEALTH QUALITY COUNCIL CHRONIC DISEASE MANAGEMENT TEAM

The Health Quality Council's Chronic Disease Management Collaborative team designed the components of this learning collaborative unique to Saskatchewan and implemented its activities. The team has been led by program directors Bonnie Brossart, Maureen Bingham, and Karen Barber. Assistant directors on this project provided assistance to collaborative facilitators and their teams in each region. They include Lisa Clatney, Helena Klomp, Sinead McGartland, Sarah Oosman, Katherine Stevenson, Tanya Verrall, Erin Walling, and Debra Woods. The lead for design of the evaluation of the collaborative is Tanya Verrall. The development and implementation of the web-based CDM

Toolkit was led by Bonnie Brossart, Katherine Stevenson, Alex Agnew, Catherine Flegel, and Pete Welch. Shari Furniss had lead responsibility for development of communications materials and the *Saskatchewan Chronic Disease Management Handbook*. Meghan Jones was responsible for logistics and administration. Dr. Vino Padayachee served as clinical chair for the collaborative, and clinical leads were Dr. Tessa Laubscher for diabetes, Dr. Mark Cameron for coronary artery disease, and Dr. Carla Eisenhauer for clinical office redesign.

NOTE

1. For readers more familiar with the terminology used in collaboratives run by the Institute for Healthcare Improvement, these individuals can be considered "faculty."

REFERENCES

Asch, S., Baker, D., Keesey, J., Broder, M., Schonlau, M., Rosen, M., et al. (2005). Does the collaborative model improve care for chronic heart failure? *Medical Care, 43,* 667-675.

Balas, E., & Boren, S. (2000). Managing clinical knowledge for health care improvement. In *Yearbook of medical informatics 2000: Patient-centered systems* (pp. 65-70). Stuttgart, Germany: Schattauer.

Centre for Chronic Disease Prevention and Control. (2002). Chapter 2 – Prevalence and incidence. In *Diabetes in Canada* (2nd ed., pp. 25-29). Ottawa, ON: Health Canada, Population and Public Health Branch.

Chan, B., Brossart, B., Hudema, N., Stevenson, K., Walling, E., Basky, G., et al. (2004). *Improving the quality of heart attack care in Saskatchewan: Outcomes and secondary prevention.* Saskatoon, SK: Health Quality Council.

Chan, B., Klomp, H., Cascagnette, P., & Brossart, B. (2006). *Quality of diabetes management in Saskatchewan.* Saskatoon, SK: Health Quality Council.

Daniel, D., Norman, J., Davis, C., Lee, H., Hindmarsh, M., McCullock, D., et al. (2004). A state-level application of the chronic illness breakthrough series: Results from two collaboratives on diabetes in Washington State. *The Joint Commission Journal on Quality and Patient Safety, 30,* 69-79.

Health Quality Council. (2005). *Saskatchewan chronic disease management handbook.* Saskatoon, SK: Author.

Heart and Stroke Foundation of Canada. (2003). *The growing burden of heart disease and stroke in Canada 2003.* Ottawa, ON: Author.

Institute for Healthcare Improvement. (2003). *The breakthrough series: IHI's collaborative model for achieving breakthrough improvement.* Boston: Author.

Langley, G., Nolan, K., Nolan, W., Norman, C., & Provost, L. (1996). Testing a change. In *The improvement guide: A practical approach to enhancing organizational performance.* (1st ed., pp. 92-112). San Francisco, CA: Jossey-Bass.

McGlynn, E., Asch, S., Adams, J., Keesey, J., Hicks, J., DeCristofaro, A., et al. (2003). The quality of health care delivered to adults in the United States. *New England Journal of Medicine, 348,* 2633-2645.

Osei, W., & Hawkey, J. (2003). *Saskatchewan diabetes profile 1996/97 to 2000/01.* Regina, SK: Saskatchewan Health.

Rogers, E. (1995). *Diffusion of innovations* (4th ed.). New York: Free Press.

Scott, I.A., Darwin, I.C., Harvey, K.H., Duke, A.B., Buckmaster, N.D., Atherton, J., Harden, H., & Ward, M. for the CHI Cardiac Collaborative. (2004). Multisite, quality-improvement collaboration to optimise cardiac care in Queensland public hospitals. *Medical Journal of Australia, 180,* 392-397.

Strategic Policy Directorate. (2002). *Economic burden of illness in Canada 1998.* Ottawa, ON: Health Canada, Population and Public Health Branch.

Wagner, E.H., Glasgow, R.E., Davis, C., Bonomi, A.E., Provost, L., McCulloch, D., Carver, P., & Sixta, C. (2001). Quality improvement in chronic illness care: A collaborative approach. *Joint Commission Journal on Quality Improvement, 27,* 63-80.

8. THE CHRONIC DISEASE SELF-MANAGEMENT PROGRAM IN BRITISH COLUMBIA

Patrick McGowan

MESH HEADINGS
British Columbia
Chronic disease
Disease management
Patient education
Self-care

BACKGROUND

In 2003 the British Columbia Ministry of Health provided health transition funding to the Centre on Aging at the University of Victoria to implement the Stanford Chronic Disease Self-Management Program (CDSMP) for a 3-year period. As the province was using the Chronic Care Model to guide service delivery, the CDSMP was considered an effective way to provide "self-management support" to people with chronic health conditions. In addition, it was a well-established and well-evaluated program that had been operating in British Columbia on a smaller scale since the late 1980s.

Self-management often means different things to different people—and sometimes different things at different times even to the same people. To date there is no "gold standard," universally accepted definition of self-management. Rather, several terms are used, sometimes interchangeably, depending on the context and focus of the discussion. These terms include self-management preparation/training, patient empowerment, and self-care. Although meant to describe a similar phenomenon, the terms imply varying specification regarding attributes, roles and responsibilities of both people with chronic health conditions and health care providers.

To illustrate the scope of related concepts, self-management is said to take place when the individual participates in treatment or in a certain type of education, such as interdisciplinary group education based on principles of adult learning, individualized treatment, and case-management theory. Others have defined self-management as a treatment intended to bring about specific outcomes—"a treatment that combines biological, psychological and social intervention techniques, with a goal of maximal functioning of regulatory processes" (Nakagawa-Kogan, Garber, Jarrett, Egan, & Hendershot, 1988, p. 105).

Redman (2004) defines self-management preparation as referring to the

> training that people with chronic health conditions need to be able to deal with taking medicine and maintaining therapeutic regimes, maintaining everyday life such as employment and family, and dealing with the future, including changing life plans and the frustration, anger, and depression. (p. 4)

Similarly, Lorig (1993) defines self-management as "learning and practicing skills necessary to carry on an active and emotionally satisfying life in the face of a chronic condition" (p. 11). Lorig further emphasizes that self-management is not an alternative to medical care. Rather, it is "aimed at helping the participant become an active, not adversarial, partner with health care providers" (p. 11).

The Expert Patient Approach (United Kingdom, National Health Service, 2001) uses the term self-management to refer to "any formalized patient education programme aimed at providing the patient with the information and skills necessary to manage their condition within the parameters of the medical regime" (p. 22). Further, these programs "are based on developing the confidence and motivation of the patient to use their own skills, information and professional services to take effective control over life with a chronic condition" (p. 22).

Self-management is said to take place when the individual engages in particular behaviours that control or reduce the impact of disease in collaboration with health care providers. Self-management is understood as

> the day-to-day tasks an individual must undertake to control or reduce the impact of disease on physical health status. At-home management tasks and strategies are undertaken with the collaboration and guidance of the individual's physician and other health care providers. (Clark, Becker, Janz, Lorig, Rakowski, & Anderson, 1991, p. 5)

Alternatively, self-management has been defined as practising specific behaviours and having the ability to reduce the physical and emotional impact of illness, regardless of the degree to which the individual participates in an education/treatment program or the type of education/treatment received. Gruman and Von Korff (1996) write that "the individual engages in activities that protect and promote health, monitors and manages symptoms and signs of illness, manages the impacts of illness on functioning, emotions and interpersonal relationships and adheres to treatment regimens" (p. 1). Glasgow, Wilson, and McCaul (1985) use the term self-management to describe the cluster of daily behaviours that patients perform to manage their chronic condition. In a similar vein, Barlow, Wright, Sheasby, Turner, and Hainsworth (2002) refer to self-management as individuals' abilities to care for themselves, regardless of how these abilities were acquired, and they do not specify a relationship with health care providers:

> Self-management refers to the individual's ability to manage the symptoms, treatment, physical and psychosocial consequences and life style changes inherent in living with a chronic condition. Efficacious self-management encompasses ability to monitor one's condition and to effect the cognitive, behavioral and emotional responses necessary to maintain a satisfactory quality of life. Thus, a dynamic and continuous process of self-regulation is established. (p. 178)

As illustrated, self-management has been defined as

- participating in education or treatment designed to bring about specific outcomes,
- preparing people to manage their health condition on a day-to-day basis,
- practising specific behaviours, and
- having the skills and abilities to reduce the physical and emotional impact of illness with or without the collaboration of the health care team.

THE PROGRAM

DEFINITION OF SELF-MANAGEMENT

As shown above, defining self-management is strategic within different contexts, and therefore one needs specificity in usage. In British Columbia, we found the definition provided by Adams, Greiner, and Corrigan (2004, p. 57) to be most helpful: "Self-management relates to the tasks that an individual must undertake to live well with one or more chronic conditions. These tasks include gaining confidence to deal with medical management, role management, and emotional management." This definition envisions self-management as behaviours, but includes the notion of "confidence" and embraces medical management (a primary concern of health care providers) as well as role and emotional management by the individual. It provides greater clarity in that the definition focuses on the person with the chronic condition. Adams et al. build on this definition in their concept of "self-management support," which specifies what health care providers can do to encourage self-management.

> Self-management support is defined as the systematic provision of education and supportive interventions by health care staff to increase patients' skills and confidence in managing their health problems, including regular assessment of progress and problems, goal setting, and problem-solving support. (p. 57)

By articulating *self-management* as behaviours and confidence to deal with medical, role, and emotional management and by using the term *self-management support* to describe what health care providers can do to facilitate it, Adams et al. have brought greater clarity to the picture.

Another factor supporting the decision to use this definition of self-management is that it is congruent with the concept of "self-management support" incorporated into the Chronic Care Model (Wagner, Austin, & Von Korff, 1996). The model was implemented through the Chronic Illness Breakthrough Series conducted by the U.S. Institute for Healthcare Improvement (Wagner, 1998). In British Columbia, the model has been modified and re-named the Expanded Chronic Care Model (Barr et al., 2003).

The model involves two overlapping realms, the community and the health care system, with self-management support as one of the four essential components within the health care system. The component "Self-Management/Develop Personal Skills" refers to "the support of self-management in coping with a disease, but also to the development of personal skills for health and wellness" (Barr et al., 2003, p. 77). Ultimately, the model posits that when "informed, activated patients" interact with a "prepared, proactive, practice team," the result is improved "functional and clinical outcomes" (see Figure 3.1). To encourage these outcomes, health authorities provide inputs to strengthen and maximize the efficiency of each component—including self-management support.

Using the definition of self-management developed by Adams et al. (2004), the goal of self-management training/education is that people will have the confidence to deal with the medical management, role management, and emotional management of their condition. To achieve this goal, the training should teach people ways to:

- access the information they seek;
- ensure they are proficient in carrying out both medically related behaviours (e.g., insulin injection, using an inhaler) and nonmedically related behaviours (e.g., interacting with their doctor, exercising);
- enhance their levels of confidence (i.e., perceived self-efficacy) in their ability to engage in these behaviours; and
- ensure they are proficient in problem-solving.

Self-management training can take place on a one-to-one basis between the individual and his or her health care provider, and in group settings led by either health providers or lay persons. This training should encourage people to identify problems, figure out barriers and supports, generate solutions, and develop long- and short-term goals (i.e., an action plan). Ways to monitor and assess progress (e.g., personal contact, telephone, mail, email) toward reaching goals need to be developed, and if the person is not successful, the problem-solving process can be repeated and new or adjusted short-term goals can be developed.

THE PROGRAM MODEL

The Chronic Disease Self-Management Program originated at the Stanford University Patient Education Research Center. Self-management education emerged as a paradigm shift in response to the aging population, increase in prevalence of chronic illness, and resulting increases in health care costs. The goal of self-management programs is to teach people general lifestyle skills needed to live with chronic health conditions and to motivate, increase confidence, and provide problem-solving abilities to manage health conditions. The CDSMP provides education on different methods of self-management through the following content: how to develop an exercise program, cognitive symptom management, nutrition management, breathing exercises, problem solving, communication skills (with family, friends, and health care providers), use of medication, and how to deal with the emotions of chronic illness such as anger and depression. The CDSMP does not take the place of traditional doctor-patient or professional-patient education but is complementary to and reinforces such education. Participants obtain new information, learn new skills and abilities, and develop higher levels of self-efficacy to manage and cope with chronic health conditions. As well, participants realize that they are not alone and the difficulties that each of them is experiencing are normal. The sessions are highly interactive, with emphasis on strategies to help individuals manage more effectively. Skills mastery is accomplished through weekly contracting to do specific behaviours and through feedback, and modelling is accomplished by lay leaders with chronic conditions and through frequent group problem-solving sessions.

The work of Albert Bandura has made a significant contribution to the field of patient self-management, particularly by articulating strategies and techniques that influence beliefs in people's capabilities to engage in behaviours. Bandura defined self-efficacy as "people's judgments of their capabilities to organize and execute courses of action required to attain designated types of performances" (1986, p. 391). The key contentions regarding the role of self-efficacy beliefs in human functioning are that "people's level of motivation, affective states, and actions are based more on what they believe than on what is objectively true" (Bandura, 1997, p. 2). The process of developing long- and short-term goals is known as "Guided Mastery." It serves as the major means for developing and expanding behavioural competencies (Bandura, 1986), and is an effective technique for raising individuals' self-efficacy. Findings from diverse lines of research reveal that perceived self-efficacy affects every phase of health behaviour change—whether people even consider changing their health behaviours, how much they benefit from treatment programs, how well they maintain the changes they have achieved, and their vulnerability to relapse. Evidence also exists that self-efficacy mediates the effects of psychosocial programs on health status (O'Leary, Shoor, Lorig, & Holman, 1988; Bandura, 2000).

Self-Management versus Patient Education

One aspect of "self-management support" (Adams et al., 2004) focuses on the educational strategies and techniques used by health professionals and lay persons. Within this area, the distinction between the type of patient education delivered by health professionals and educators is sometimes blurred with what is known as self-management education. Both types of education are essential in assisting the individual achieve the best quality of life and independence; the intent here is to compare and contrast their attributes.

In some instances, self-management education has been defined as meaning the same as patient education. For example, Clement (1995) argued that "the term self-management education emphasizes the need for people with diabetes to manage their diabetes on a day-to-day basis. For this reason the terms *diabetes education* and *self-management education* will refer to the same process" (p. 1204). Therefore, Clement considered "treatment behaviours," which are the major focus of traditional patient education, to be synonymous with self-management behaviours because it was the individual (i.e., the self) who would practise them. Treatment behaviours for diabetes include self-injection of insulin, self-monitoring of glucose levels, eating properly, smoking cessation, exercising, and taking medications properly. By practising these behaviours there is an expectation that intermediate goals will be achieved (i.e., metabolic control, optimal blood glucose levels, blood lipid control, and achieving and maintaining a healthy weight). And, if these intermediate goals are achieved, there should be better diabetes outcomes: a reduction in morbidity (retinopathy, neuropathy, nephropathy), fewer hospitalizations, a reduction in diabetes-related health care costs, and reduced mortality. One cannot minimize the benefits of this type of education, whether it is referred to as patient education or self-management education, in that there is strong evidence linking these behaviours to diabetes outcomes (Corabian & Harstall, 2001; Peyrot, 1999; McLeod, 1998; Brown et al., 1996; Brown, 1992; Brown, 1990; Brown, 1988; Padgett, Mumford, Hynes, & Carter, 1988).

More recently, the major differences between patient education and self-management education have been delineated by Bodenheimer, Lorig, Holman, and Grumbach (2002). Traditional patient education provides information and teaches technical disease-related skills, whereas self-management education teaches skills on how to act on problems.

- Problems covered in traditional patient education reflect widespread common problems related to a specific disease, whereas the problems covered in self-management education are identified by the patient.
- Traditional patient education is disease-specific and offers information and technical skills related to the disease. In comparison, self-management education provides problem-solving skills that are relevant to the consequences of chronic conditions in general.
- Traditional patient education is based on the underlying theory that disease-specific knowledge creates behaviour change, which in turn produces better outcomes. Self-management education, in contrast, is based on the theory that greater patient confidence in his/her capacity to make life-improving changes yields better clinical outcomes.
- The goal of traditional patient education is "compliance," whereas the goal in self-management education is increased self-efficacy and improved clinical outcomes.

• In traditional patient education the health professional is the educator, but in self-management education the educators may be health professionals, peer leaders, or other patients.

Implementation During 2003–2006

The Chronic Disease Self-Management Program trains lay people who have chronic health conditions to lead weekly sessions for 6 weeks in their local communities. Two leaders deliver each course. Some leaders may have other leadership roles in their communities through health, cultural, political, or religious organizations. The use of community volunteer leaders not only reduces the need for expensive professional personnel, it also strengthens the education. Community people serve as influential role models for promoting self-management skills and self-efficacy. Considering the growing prevalence of chronic health conditions and the limited number of health professionals, the use of a group format with community volunteer leaders is highly cost effective. As program leaders are community residents, they are in a good position to encourage participation of others who normally do not participate in community programs.

To lead the Chronic Disease Self-Management Program, persons must successfully complete a 4-day leader-training workshop delivered by two certified master trainers. Up to 18 participants learn how to use the Leader's Manual to deliver the course. The manual consists of a scripted protocol for the six sessions, which must be delivered as specified. Each weekly session consists of five to six activities. During the leader-training workshop, each activity is demonstrated by the master trainers and then discussed with trainees. This training includes participating in and discussing all aspects of the intervention, extensive practice teaching, and learning to deal with problems that arise in small groups. As well, trainees demonstrate that they can follow the Leader's Manual by conducting two practice teaching sessions. The master trainers evaluate each trainee and provide certificates to those who demonstrate that they can follow the Leader's Manual to deliver the course. The leader-training workshops are set up by CDSMP coordinators. British Columbia has three coordinators who liaise with health professionals and lay persons in the health regions to identify key contact persons who assist setting up a workshop.

Experience over a 10-year period has shown that approximately 50% of trained leaders actually deliver the CDSMP course. Approximately 10% exceed this commitment and lead additional courses as well. When people agree to become leaders, they give a verbal commitment that they will lead two Chronic Disease Self-Management Program courses during the next year. However, about half of the participants are unable to fulfil this commitment because of worsening illness, changing family situation, severe weather conditions, personal travel, difficulty registering participants (smaller communities can only support one or two courses), and getting another leader to work with them. Another consideration is that small communities can realistically deliver the

CDSMP only a few times a year, therefore involving only a few leaders. For instance, if 12 leaders are trained in a community, only six to eight may have an opportunity to deliver the program; however, all leaders receive the benefit of the 4-day workshop.

The trained leaders then deliver the Chronic Disease Self-Management Program to groups of 10 to 12 people once each week for 2½ hours for 6 consecutive weeks in community settings (senior centres, libraries, hospitals, and recreation centres). Course participants are persons who are experiencing chronic health conditions, and their significant others. Each participant in the workshop receives a copy of the companion book, the Canadian version of *Living a Healthy Life with Chronic Conditions, 2nd Edition* (Lorig et al., 2004).

CDSMP coordinators assist leaders to set up courses. The leaders are requested to find suitable locations, advertise the course, register 10 to 12 interested persons, and prepare a set of course flipcharts. The coordinator provides assistance with these tasks and sends brochures, posters, "canned" newspaper articles, and other helpful materials. When the leaders have a course scheduled with the adequate number of registrants, the coordinator sends the required number of course books. Leaders are also sent sign-in sheets and program evaluation questionnaires, which they distribute and collect. When the course is completed, the leaders send the sign-in sheets and evaluations to the program coordinator. The coordinator then sends each leader a $50 honorarium. Table 8.1 shows the number of leader-training workshops, trained leaders, courses, and participants in British Columbia's five health regions. Variations may be attributed to geographic location and community size.

Table 8.1
Implementation of the Chronic Disease Self-Management Program in British Columbia, 2003–2006

Health Region	Leader-Training Workshops	Trained Leaders	No. of Courses	Participants
Vancouver Island	11	118	79	827
Vancouver Coastal	13	158	108	1,414
Fraser	9	86	61	688
Interior	17	192	101	1,087
Northern	15	152	37	352
Total	65	706	386	4,368

OUTCOMES

The CDSMP was evaluated in a randomized, controlled trial conducted by the Stanford University Patient Education Research Center (Lorig et al., 1999). In this study, effectiveness was measured in terms of changes in behaviour, health status, and health service utilization. Data were collected at two points 6 months apart by mailed questionnaires from 952 patients (all over age 40), of whom 561 were randomly assigned to the treatment group and 391 to the control group. There were no significant differences in baseline data between the treatment and control groups.

Health behaviour changes occurred more often in the treatment group than in the control group for all three behaviour-change indicators: number of minutes per week of exercise, increased practice of cognitive symptom management, and improved communication with their physician. Treatment group subjects also had more positive scores for self-rated health status, including disability, social/role activity limitation, energy/fatigue, and health distress. Finally, fewer hospital admissions and fewer nights in hospital were found for the treatment group. No significant differences in visits to physicians were identified, however.

In a 2-year post-program follow-up study (Lorig et al., 2001), the researchers found that compared with baseline for each of the 2 years, emergency room and outpatient visits, and health distress were reduced ($p < .05$), and self-efficacy improved ($p < .05$). Further dissemination studies conducted by Kaiser Permanente found similar results. In British Columbia, 8 evaluation studies were conducted between 1992 and 2002. Using the same outcome measures as Stanford University and a one-group pre- and six-month post-program design, results showed improvements in self-efficacy (8 studies), pain level (6 studies), health status (5 studies), depression (4 studies), level of stress and disability (4 studies).

Between April 1, 2003, and March 31, 2006, nearly 700 program participants completed pre- and six-month post-program questionnaires. This analysis involved a pre- and six-month post-program matched-group comparison of outcome measures. The majority of persons (83%) indicated that English was their mother tongue, 52% were married or living with a partner, and 60% had more than one chronic health condition. The most common health condition was arthritis or other rheumatic disease. Participant ages ranged from 15 to 93 years with the average being 58 years ($SD = 14$). The mean education level was 14 years ($SD = 3$). Eighty-two percent of participants were female.

Health measure scores were computed and compared between the two time periods to calculate whether differences were statistically significant. Changes were observed on 14 of the 16 outcome measures. At six-months post-program, participants were using more coping strategies to deal with pain or symptoms; were communicating more with their physician (preparing written questions, asking questions, discussing problems); were spending more time doing aerobic exercise; had higher self-efficacy in their ability to manage disease symptoms; had higher self-efficacy in their ability to manage their disease; perceived they were in better health; had less disability (dressing, arising, eating, walking, hygiene, reaching, gripping, activities); felt their disease had less of an impact on social and recreational activities; were experiencing fewer depressive symptoms; had more energy and less fatigue; were experiencing less distress; were experiencing less fatigue; were experiencing less pain; and felt the disease had a lesser impact on their lives. This evaluation did not include the analysis of health care utilization. This particular aspect of the program is currently being planned and results will be available in 2007.

LESSONS LEARNED

Norris, Engelgau, and Venkat Narayan (2001) systematically reviewed 72 reports of published randomized controlled trials conducted since 1980 examining the effectiveness of patient education. In their conclusion, Norris et al. noted that criteria for ideal self-management interventions should include the following conditions: behavioural interventions must be practical and feasible in a variety of settings; a large percentage of the relevant population must be willing to participate; the intervention must be effective for long-term important physiological outcomes, behavioural end points, and quality of life; patients must be satisfied; and the program must be relatively low cost and cost-effective.

The 3-year experience in British Columbia shows that the CDSMP has met these criteria; however, there continues to be other ongoing challenges facing the program. The first challenge relates to the definition of patient self-management. The term continues to be used to mean different things and, to further this confusion, published meta-analysis studies that examine effectiveness use broad and nonspecific terminology and meanings. The second challenge relates to the program's integration with traditional patient education, which has only been attempted in a few locations. It appears that this type of coordination and the additional work for health professionals to work with volunteer leaders is challenging. The third challenge relates to interactions between "informed, activated patients" and the "prepared, proactive practice team." There is no point in training people with chronic health conditions to be confident and proactive in their care if the practice team does not share this philosophy.

The fourth challenge is that the self-management programs appear to be operating at arm's length from primary care physicians. Attempts to develop pathways where patients are instructed by physicians to take the CDSMP course have been futile. Patients generally follow physician requests regarding lab tests and X-rays, but not regarding patient education, which appears to be a problem across the spectrum of care. While this may be considered problematic, it may merely reflect the way that things happen in real life. For example, most care providers would agree that it is more advantageous to interact with patients when they are motivated and ready to change. However, the current policy and procedure reflects a different sequence, which is not supported by Stages of Change theory—Symptoms → Diagnosis → Education → Treatment.

With the self-management program, people register when they are ready, when they acknowledge that they are experiencing difficulties and problems in their everyday lives and are motivated to do something about it. People who register for self-management frequently say that they had known about the program for a few years and did not feel they needed it, but now they do. For some reason people with chronic health conditions take the initiative to register—in British Columbia, 5,805 people registered between 2000 and 2006.

As well, studies have shown that offering the program on a continual basis with varying schedules over a 20-year period encouraged participation, as approximately 40% of a closed cohort of persons with chronic illness attended (Bruce, Lorig, & Laurent, 2005).

ACKNOWLEDGEMENT

Implementation of the Chronic Disease Self-Management Program throughout British Columbia is due in large part to the vision and foresight of Valerie Tregillus, Executive Director, Primary Health Care, Medical Services Division, BC Ministry of Health.

REFERENCES

Adams, K., Greiner, A.C., & Corrigan, J.M. (Eds.). (2004). *Report of a summit. The 1st annual crossing the quality chasm summit—A focus on communities.* Washington: National Academies Press.

Bandura, A. (1986). *Social foundations of thought and action: A social cognitive theory.* Englewood Cliff, NJ: Prentice-Hall.

Bandura, A. (1997). *Self-Efficacy: The exercise of control.* New York: W.H. Freeman and Company.

Bandura, A. (2000). Self-Efficacy: The foundation of agency. In W.J. Perrig (Ed.), *Control of human behaviour, mental processes and consciousness* (pp. 17-33). Mahwah, NJ: Lawrence Erlbaum.

Barlow, J., Wright, C., Sheasby, J., Turner, A., & Hainsworth, J. (2002). Self-management approaches for people with chronic conditions: A review. *Patient Education and Counseling, 48,* 177-187.

Barr, V.J., Robinson, S., Marin-Link, B., Underhill, L., Dotts, A., Ravensdale, D., & Salivaras, S. (2003). The Expanded Chronic Care Model: An integration of concepts and strategies from population health promotion and the chronic care model. *Hospital Quarterly, 7*(1), 73-81.

Bodenheimer, T., Lorig, K., Holman, H., & Grumbach, K. (2002). Patient self-management of chronic disease in primary care. *Journal of the American Medical Association, 288*(19), 2469-2475.

Brown, S. (1988). Effects of educational interventions in diabetes care: A meta-analysis of findings. *Nursing Research, 37,* 223-230.

Brown, S. (1990). Studies of educational interventions and outcomes in diabetic adults: A meta-analysis revisited. *Patient Education & Counseling, 16*(3), 189-215.

Brown S.A. (1992). Meta-analysis of diabetes patient education research: Variations in intervention effects across studies. *Research in Nursing & Health, 15*(6), 409-419.

Brown S.A., Upchurch, S., Arding, R., Winter, M., & Ramirez, G. (1996). Promoting weight loss in type 2 diabetes. *Diabetes Care, 19*(6), 613-624.

Bruce, B., Lorig, K., & Laurent, D. (2005, September). *If you bug them, they will come: Participation in self-management programs in a cohort of arthritis patients.* Paper presented at New Perspectives Conference, Victoria, BC.

Clark, N.M., Becker, M.H., Janz, N.K., Lorig, K., Rakowski, W., & Anderson, L. (1991). Self-management of chronic disease by older adults. A review and questions for older adults. *Journal of Aging and Health, 3,* 3-27.

Clement, S. (1995). Diabetes self-management education. *Diabetes Care, 18*(8), 1204-1214.

Corabian, P., & Harstall, C. (2001). *Patient diabetes education in the management of type 2 diabetes.* Alberta Heritage Foundation for Medical Research, HA 23: Series A, Health Technology Assessment.

Glasgow, R.E., Wilson, W., & McCaul, K.D. (1985). Regimen adherence: A problematic construct in diabetes research. *Diabetes Care, 8,* 300-301.

Gruman, J., & Von Korff, M. (1996). *Indexed bibliography on self-management for people with chronic disease.* Washington: Center for Advancement in Health.

Lorig, K. (1993). Self-management of chronic illness: A model for the future. *Generations, XVII*(3), 11-14.

Lorig, K., Holman, H., Sobel, D., Laurent, D., Gonzalez, V., Minor, M., & McGowan, P. (2004). *Living a healthy life with chronic conditions* (Canadian ed.). Colorado: Bull Publishing.

Lorig, K.R., Ritter, P., Stewart, A.L., Sobel, D.S., Brown, B.W., Bandura, A., Gonzalez, V.M., Laurent, D.D., & Holman, H.R. (2001). Chronic Disease Self-Management Program: 2-year health status and health care utilization outcomes. *Medical Care, 39*(11), 1217-1223.

Lorig, K., Sobel, D., Stewart, A., Brown, W., Bandura, A., Ritter, P., Gonzalez, V., Laurent, D., & Holman, H. (1999). Evidence suggesting that a chronic disease self-management program can improve health status while reducing hospitalization—A randomized trial. *Medical Care, 37*(1), 5-14.

Nakagawa-Kogan, H., Garber, A., Jarrett, M., Egan, K.J., & Hendershot, S. (1988). Self-management of hypertension: Predictors of success in diastolic blood pressure reduction. *Research in Nursing & Health, 11,* 105-115.

McLeod, B. (1998). Research in diabetes education: Where have we been and where do we want to go? *Canadian Journal of Diabetes Care, 22*(2), 20-28.

Norris, S., Engelgau, M., & Venkat Narayan, K. (2001). Effectiveness of self-management training in type 2 diabetes. *Diabetes Care, 24*(3), 561-587.

O'Leary, A., Shoor, S., Lorig, K., & Holman, H.R. (1988). A cognitive-behavioral treatment for rheumatoid arthritis. *Health Psychology, 7*(6), 527-544.

Padgett, D., Mumford, E., Hynes, M., & Carter, R. (1988). Meta-analysis of the effects of educational and psychosocial interventions on the management of diabetes mellitus. *Journal of Clinical Epidemiology, 41,* 1007-1030.

Peyrot, M. (1999). Behavior change in diabetes education. *Diabetes Educator, 25*(65), 62-73.

Redman, B.K. (2004). *Patient self-management of chronic disease: The health care provider's challenge.* Sudbury, MA: Jones & Bartlett Publishers.

United Kingdom. National Health Service. (2001). *The expert patient: A new approach to chronic disease management for the 21st century.* London, UK: Department of Health.

Wagner, E., Austin, B., & Von Korff, M. (1996). Organizing care for patients with chronic illness. *Millbank Quarterly, 74*(4), 511-544.

9. GETTING A GRIP ON ARTHRITIS: A NATIONAL PRIMARY HEALTH CARE COMMUNITY INITIATIVE

Sydney Lineker, Mary J. Bell, Jennifer Boyle, and Elizabeth Badley

MESH HEADINGS
Arthritis
Canada
Chronic disease
Disease management
Education, medical continuing
Ontario
Patient care team
Patient education
Primary health care

BACKGROUND

In 1999, a successful educational model, Getting a Grip on Arthritis, was developed and piloted in Ontario (Glazier, Badley, Lineker, Wilkins, & Bell, 2005), with funding from the Ontario Ministry of Health and Long-term Care. It was one of the first to show changes in the management of arthritis in a primary health care setting. The intervention increased awareness of arthritis best practices for both people with arthritis and providers, and improved provider confidence in managing arthritis. The pilot project also demonstrated a practical approach to the implementation and dissemination of clinical practice guidelines in a primary health care environment, which may serve as a model for other chronic diseases. Collaboration between the various members of the primary health care team (physicians, nurses, nurse practitioners, health promoters, and others) and the person with arthritis was a key to the success of the intervention. As a result, an application was submitted to Health Canada's Primary Health Care Transition Fund and, in 2004–2005, support was received to implement the program nationally.

Why should arthritis be a priority? Arthritis is a leading cause of disability, and costs Canadians over $4 billion in health care and lost work days annually.

Arthritis is one of the leading reasons for physician visits (over 9 million visits per year), clearly demonstrating the need for appropriate diagnosis and management at the primary care level. Previous work has demonstrated that there are multiple barriers to appropriate care delivery for people with arthritis. In particular, physicians report difficulties in diagnosing rheumatoid arthritis and delays in referral to specialists; patients report lack of information on medications, side effects, and self-management strategies.

THE PROGRAM

The Getting a Grip on Arthritis project was a joint initiative involving a partnership between The Arthritis Society and eight other organizations with the goal of implementing best practices for osteoarthritis and rheumatoid arthritis in primary health care settings across Canada. Partners included The Arthritis Society, Sunnybrook Health Sciences Centre, Canadian Alliance of Community Health Centre Associations, Canadian Nurses Association, Arthritis Community Research and Evaluation Unit, Canadian Rheumatology Association, Arthritis Health Professions Association, Patient Partners® in Arthritis, and the Ontario Ministry of Health and Long-term Care.

The project was administered by The Arthritis Society out of its head office in Toronto. Thirteen staff worked out of offices in Toronto, Vancouver, Regina, Sudbury, Montreal, and St. John's. The Arthritis Community Research and Evaluation Unit was responsible for project evaluation. All project staff had access to a team room for sharing and archiving documents.

The aims of the national project were to increase the capacity of primary health care providers, communities, and people with arthritis to manage the burden of arthritis, and to evaluate the implementation of a national community-based educational project designed to improve the diagnosis and treatment of arthritis in primary care (guideline implementation). The program was based on social learning theory and used strategies known to influence provider behaviour change: opportunities for networking and team building, demonstration and practice, hands-on skill development, reinforcement, evaluation, peer models, goal setting, and incentives. The educational intervention focused on individual health professionals, their work environment, and their community. It included three components: educational resources for patients and providers, workshops, and reinforcement activities.

EDUCATIONAL RESOURCES

These materials were revised versions of those developed as part of the original Getting a Grip on Arthritis project in Ontario, and were based on patient and health provider input and evidence available through published arthritis guidelines. Materials were developed in French and English. A poster focusing on primary and secondary prevention messages was created based on a literature search on prevention and arthritis. One article provided an excellent summary of the literature (Rao & Hootman, 2004) and these primary messages were used in the poster. A secondary prevention message (Do you have arthritis?) was added to the poster to encourage people who have early symptoms of arthritis to see their physician.

Provider educational material included arthritis textbooks, a prescription pad to prompt appropriate referrals, and a laminated pocket card summarizing arthritis best practices identified in a review of current literature.

Patient educational material included a Resource Kit, arthritis books, and videos for each participating primary health care site. The kit provides information on the roles of primary health care team members, and on best practices for osteoarthritis and rheumatoid arthritis as identified in the literature and selected resources (books, videos, websites). A province-specific section (Financial and Other Resources for People with Arthritis) was created. Efforts were made to ensure that the Resource Kit was easy to read and understand. The kit was then assessed using the Flesch-Kincaid Grade Level available in MS Word, which indicated that reading levels ranged from grade 6.2 for the section on surgery to grade 12 for the sections on financial resources and recommended reading. The Resource Kit was also made available in cassette and CD format for those who could not read due to limited vision or literacy.

WORKSHOP DESIGN AND DELIVERY

Workshop design and content were based on arthritis best practices developed through the pilot study and updated through a review of the literature. Eligible primary health care sites across Canada were identified through a number of sources including partner organizations and Ministry of Health representatives. As well, stakeholder meetings were held in each province to help determine appropriate and interested participants. A letter of invitation was sent to the executive director of each prospective organization outlining the project and the benefits of participating. All health care providers who educated or treated people with arthritis at sites that volunteered to participate were then invited to register for a workshop in their community or region. When space was available, health care providers from local hospitals, home care agencies, and other health care facilities were invited to attend.

Workshop attendance, content and faculty reflected the interprofessional model of care. Content focused on best practices for the primary care management of osteoarthritis and rheumatoid arthritis, and included evidence-based pharmacological and nonpharmacological interventions (education, psychosocial support, exercise, weight management/nutrition, assistive devices, and joint protection). Faculty included 249 multidisciplinary health professionals (rheumatologists, pharmacists, occupational therapists, physiotherapists, social workers, dietitians) as well as Arthritis Self-Management Program leaders and 94 trained patient educators. The session with patients provided participants with an opportunity to enhance their musculoskeletal examination skills.

The workshops were unique in that the team of health professionals from each participating site was invited to attend along with local arthritis specialists. At the end of the workshop, participants from each community met in small groups to plan how to implement arthritis best practices in their community.

REINFORCEMENT ACTIVITIES

The objectives of the reinforcement activities were to strengthen the messages on arthritis best practices delivered in the workshops, and to support the delivery of integrated arthritis care in the community. Reinforcement activities were defined as follows:

- Primary—activities and information offered to all sites during the reinforcement time frame following the workshop (e.g., newsletters, books, videos, resource lists);
- Secondary—activities requested by sites during the reinforcement time frame (e.g., Arthritis Self-Management Program leadership training, advanced arthritis education, equipment); and
- Tertiary—reinforcement activities to support the delivery of arthritis care in the community and not specific to a primary health care site (e.g., provincial events, faculty requests for educational materials).

Only those activities that were funded by the project are summarized in this report. Other unfunded reinforcement activities also may have taken place (e.g., the provision of information, linking people with resources). All participating sites received at least one form of primary reinforcement.

OUTCOMES

HIGH PARTICIPATION RATE/REACH

Over 430 primary health care organizations were invited to participate, and 219 sent participants to the workshops. Thirty workshops on arthritis best practices (24 English, 6 French) were delivered to 900 health care providers in rural and urban communities in 10 provinces between September 2004 and November 2005. Objectives of the workshops were for providers to understand arthritis clinical practice guidelines and ways to improve the delivery of arthritis care, to review/improve their musculoskeletal physical examination skills, and to make a plan for local implementation of arthritis best practices.

Workshop participants included 646 primary health care providers and 254 providers working in other types of facilities including hospitals, rehab centres, home care agencies, and fee-for-service clinics. The range of participants reflected the interprofessional model of care (physicians, 15%; nurse practitioners,

11%; other health care providers, 63%; nonclinical staff/students, 10%). The primary health care providers came from a variety of organizations (community health centres, 26%; family health networks/primary care networks in Ontario, 6%; Centre de santé et service sociaux/Groupes de médecine de famille in Quebec, 18%; other primary health care organizations, 50%).

Participants were asked to complete an evaluation at the end of the workshop. Over 90% of participants found the workshops were relevant, met stated objectives, met their personal learning objectives and expectations, allowed opportunity to interact with colleagues, were credible and nonbiased, and were well organized. The most common complaint was related to the lack of adequate time allowed for the amount of content covered. Workshop sessions/speakers received positive evaluations, with the trained patient educator session rated the highest.

Participants were asked to describe two particularly strong features of the workshop and two things they would like to see improved. Strengths of the workshops included the team learning opportunity, the interactive and varied format, the involvement of people with arthritis and local faculty, the opportunity to improve their musculoskeletal examination skills and the opportunity to link with local resources. Challenges included the mixed needs of the participants and skill level of the faculty, and scope of practice issues.

We piloted one workshop with fee-for-service providers in the Owen Sound area. This workshop received the best evaluation of all our workshops, suggesting that this educational model would work successfully in a fee-for-service environment, should funding become available to deliver this program to this audience.

The workshops were accredited for nine MAINPRO-C credits by the College of Family Physicians of Canada. MAINPRO-C accreditation required that the providers complete a baseline and post-workshop survey (online or paper-based), and a reflective practice exercise during the reinforcement phase after the workshop. All non-physicians received a certificate of participation upon completion of their workshop evaluations.

REINFORCEMENT ACTIVITIES

Patient and provider books and videos were delivered to 165 sites (75%). A reflective practice exercise was sent to providers in 213 sites (97%); 58 out of 151 physicians (38%) completed the exercise and received MAINPRO-C credits. In addition, 98 non-physicians participated in this process. Providers from 191 sites (99%) received follow-up calls or emails relating to their personal goals established at the workshops. Providers from 203 sites (93%) received a copy of the arthritis resource list for their community or region, and providers at 210 sites (96%) were emailed electronic copies of the referral and consultation templates discussed at the workshop. One hundred and forty-three sites (65%) ordered educational materials for their patients or providers. The most common request was for the Resource Kit for Patients with Arthritis (26,495 copies). To support the community, arthritis books and videos were donated to 159 local libraries.

Forty-six sites (21%) requested secondary reinforcement activities. The most common requests were for PACE (Patient Assessment and Counseling for Exercise) materials (27 requests), and for additional staff training (18 requests). There were 87 tertiary reinforcement activities provided to support the delivery of arthritis best practices in the community. The most common activities were the provision of educational materials to faculty, providers at non-primary health care sites, and The Arthritis Society, and the provision of professional development activities to community clinicians. The total cost of all reinforcement activities for the project was $214,969.

EDUCATIONAL MATERIALS ONLINE

All educational materials developed for the project in French and English have been put in PDF format and are available online for free download on The Arthritis Society (2006) website.

SURVEY OF WORKSHOP FACULTY, FACILITATORS, AND GUESTS

Throughout the project, we heard many stories from our workshop faculty, facilitators, and guests indicating that they had learned so much through their participation and how they had changed their practice. We decided it would be important to capture this information and surveyed this group. We received 207 out of 377 surveys back for a response rate of 55%. Respondents reported that the greatest influence of the project was in the area of improved arthritis care in the community.

QUALITATIVE RESULTS

As a result of our project, the Centre de santé et service sociaux La Mitis has initiated a new interdisciplinary arthritis clinic in the Bas St-Laurent region with rheumatologist Dr. Fortin from Rimouski. Dr. Fortin plans to educate the family doctors on arthritis best practices including intra-articular injection skills. As well, staff from Albert County Wellness Centre who attended our workshop in Fredericton, New Brunswick, linked with Dr. Doherty in Moncton and established a new arthritis clinic.

LESSONS LEARNED

STAFF RECRUITMENT

It took 9 months to get all the staff in place, as it was critical to have the right people with the right skills. This delay affected the timelines and resulted in a staggered implementation of the project across Canada. This approach ultimately worked well, since we made adjustments to the program as it rolled out. However, it resulted in some challenges at the end of the project because the last provinces to implement the program had less time to do the follow-up activities, and evaluation timelines had to be shortened for three workshops.

ETHICS

There were significant challenges in obtaining ethics approvals for this project in multiple jurisdictions across Canada. Health Canada's ethics guidelines were not sufficient in most jurisdictions, and we had to submit over 20 ethics proposals. Patient surveying was another challenge, because in many jurisdictions patient names could not be given to the researchers. This required that we use on-site staff not familiar with survey methods and privacy requirements to handle the patient survey mailings. Additional project staff and training time were needed to ensure that we met privacy requirements.

TECHNOLOGY

The lack of computerized databases and/or appropriate coding of osteoarthritis and rheumatoid arthritis in primary health care sites to allow identification of appropriate patients resulted in fewer patients being surveyed than expected (approximately 3,400 patients were surveyed). We therefore offered some primary health care sites the opportunity to do manual chart reviews to identify patients with arthritis. Only a few sites had the time and human resources to contribute to this effort. Some sites were hesitant to agree to patient surveys due to the new privacy legislation and the extra level of staff commitment required. An electronic medical record, coding standards, and staff training would help alleviate these problems.

DIFFERENCES IN PRIMARY HEALTH CARE MODELS

Not all primary health care organizations were the same in terms of the team, type of remuneration, catchment area, target population, and health priorities. To address these differences, we defined a primary health care site quite broadly as a not-for-profit organization that served adults with arthritis and delivered primary health care services. Some organizations, like Community Health Centres, had multidisciplinary staff with a long history of working as a team and with their communities. Other organizations, especially those that were newly formed, either did not have the team in place or had staff who were not trained in how to work as a team in a community setting. It was clear that some staff were uncomfortable with their new roles in a primary health care environment. Our workshops promoted the development of community teams and allowed providers to see how they could develop skills needed in their new role in community-based chronic disease management. Where there was no team, the workshops helped build the team using existing community resources or virtual connections.

RECRUITMENT OF PARTICIPANTS

In many organizations, arthritis was not the priority, making the recruitment of providers a challenge. Some organizations chose not to participate because asthma or diabetes was their focus. We emphasized that many of the messages and skills learned in our workshops would apply to other chronic diseases (e.g., maintain a healthy weight, exercise regularly), and that the program was a model for chronic disease management using existing resources and was also an opportunity for team building.

The timing of the workshops was another factor in recruitment. In some locations, there were other training opportunities, conferences, and workshops that were competing with our program. Our stakeholders were important sources of information regarding competing programs and advised us regarding the best timing for the workshops.

POLICY

Policy level changes that would assist in program implementation relate to roles and scope of practice issues. Specifically, our workshops generated interesting discussions regarding regulations on who can diagnose, who can refer to specialists, and how specialists would be remunerated if referrals came from health professionals other than physicians. Provincial licensing issues arose when we used health professionals to teach in provinces other than where they were licensed. Scope of practice for nurse practitioners around prescribing and referrals varied in each province.

SUSTAINABILITY

Project sustainability requires infrastructure, resources, and expertise to continue to update the program content and maintain the program nationally. This has been a challenge since there is no national organization with a mandate to fund and/or train health professionals to work in an interdisciplinary manner. Workshop slide presentations have been made available to participants and faculty in the hopes that they will use these resources to train others within their organizations and communities.

ACKNOWLEDGEMENTS:

The authors would like to acknowledge the significant contributions of the staff in The Arthritis Society offices across Canada and those at the Arthritis Community Research and Evaluation Unit, who contributed significantly to the implementation and evaluation of this project. As well, we would like to thank our partners, workshop faculty, members of the Canadian rheumatology community, and the many community stakeholders who made this project possible. Special mention has to made of the 94 people with arthritis who travelled the country with us and participated as educators in our workshops.

REFERENCES

Glazier, R.H., Badley, E.M., Lineker, S.C., Wilkins, A.L., & Bell, M.J. (2005). Getting a grip on arthritis: An educational intervention for the diagnosis and treatment of arthritis in primary care. *Journal of Rheumatology 32*(1), 137-142.

Rao, J.K., & Hootman, J.M. (2004). Prevention research and rheumatic disease. *Current Opinion in Rheumatology 16*(2), 119-124.

The Arthritis Society. (2006). Getting a Grip on Arthritis project. Retrieved February 27, 2007, from http://www.arthritis.ca/programs%20and%20resources/getting%20a%20grip/default.asp?s=1

10. THE LEADER DIABETES INITIATIVE: OPTIMIZING DIABETES CARE IN SASKATCHEWAN

Mikki Millar

MESH HEADINGS
Chronic disease
Diabetes mellitus
Disease management
Health care reform
Patient care team
Patient education
Primary health care
Rural health services
Saskatchewan
Self-care

BACKGROUND

In an era of health care reform, where the challenge is to create sustainable programs for enhancing patient care, it is obvious why primary health care has quickly become the focus. The Saskatchewan government and other various health organizations have realized the potential of primary health care to prevent, diagnose, and treat chronic conditions. They are dedicated to enhancing primary care for chronic conditions by improving treatment and follow-up based on accepted practice guidelines; improving case management for clients with complex needs; introducing more proactive approaches to reach high-risk populations; ensuring that care is provided by the professionals who can best meet the needs of the client; improving screening and monitoring programs to support early detection and intervention; ensuring that health services are continuous with and complementary to other community services; and supporting and enabling self-care. The Leader Diabetes Initiative was designed to work toward achieving all of these strategies.

To understand the initiative and its challenges, some background information is necessary. Leader is located in southwest Saskatchewan, close to the Alberta border. With an estimated population of 950 people, this rural, agriculturally based town is the local hub of medical activity. The three salaried physicians and a nurse practitioner serve over 2,000 patients, including two Hutterite colonies and various surrounding villages and hamlets. Local facilities include a 20-bed hospital with limited laboratory services, a 36-bed long-term care facility, emergency medical services, and a community pharmacy. Leader is a remote community with the nearest regional hospital (in Medicine Hat, Alberta) approximately 1½ hours away, and the closest tertiary centre 3 hours away by car.

Leader and area has a slightly greater than 5% incidence of diagnosed diabetes among the local population, due in part to the high rate of diabetes in our local Hutterite population. With the health region average of diagnosed diabetes at 5%, the need for a comprehensive diabetic program was an obvious one.

The concept for the Leader Diabetes Initiative (LDI) came from the local clinical pharmacist, Charity Evans. True to the spirit of rural life, in October 2003 Evans volunteered to drive an elderly patient to the nearest diabetes education centre in Medicine Hat for a 2-day diabetes clinic. After sitting in on the clinic, she realized that with some effort and a few additional resources, the same care could be provided in the Leader area. In March 2004, Evans presented her proposal for the LDI to the local health authority, Cypress Health Region. While it was well received, funding was difficult to obtain. In August 2004, Leader was designated an official primary health care site by Saskatchewan Health, and recruitment for a nurse practitioner began. Although funding from the health region was not secured until later, Evans, with guaranteed financial support from her employer, began to proceed in January 2005. The initiative ran from March to September 2005.

Soon a database of area patients with diabetes was developed and the process of collecting baseline data began. The community pharmacist reviewed the charts and gave recommendations to the health care providers, highlighting those patients who had not reached clinical targets and adding a flow sheet to each chart. The flow sheet was copied onto coloured paper, so as to stand out in the patient's file. It included information on comorbidities, medications, referral checklist, weight, creatinine clearance, targets for pre- and postprandial glucometer values, AIC, lipid levels (LDL and ratio), and blood pressure.

Once all baseline data were collected, team development began. Members of the "core" team included the patient, three physicians, the nurse practitioner, the community pharmacist, and the dietitian. While the core members had more direct patient contact, other team members had equally important roles. These members included professionals from emergency medical services, podiatry, mental health, home care, and public health. Our remote location made team building a challenge. Many of our community services are provided by visiting professionals who come to us from Swift Current. Leader is fortunate, however, in that most of the visiting professionals have a satellite office in the same building as the medical clinic, making communication easier. Each team member was asked what they would see their role to be in the initiative. After feedback was received, an initial comprehensive meeting was held with most of the team members present. At this meeting, the mandate of the initiative was outlined. Clinical targets were communicated to all team members according to the 2003 Canadian Diabetes Association (CDA) clinical practice guidelines. Individual roles were defined, and logistics related to the use of the flow sheet and data collection were reviewed. At that time, an initial patient list and baseline data were supplied to each team member.

Much of the team development that followed the initial meeting took place informally. Core team members communicated daily through email, phone, or informal meetings in the clinic. Updated patient lists, clinical data, and graphed progress charts were given to the core team members monthly. Non-core team members received the graphed progress charts monthly and regular communications, usually via email.

Patients were informed of the initiative in various ways. Blood glucose logbooks, informational pamphlets, and a letter describing the initiative were sent out to all identified patients with diabetes. Posters with a description of the Leader Diabetes Initiative were displayed in the hospital, clinic, pharmacy, and various "coffee spots" around the area. The medical providers also played a large role in the initiation phase. They explained the Leader Diabetes Initiative in detail to every patient with diabetes, and invited the patient to sign a consent form allowing all team members access to appropriate information in his or her file. The decision to participate or opt out of the initiative was the first step in including the patient in the decision-making process.

THE PROGRAM

The initiative focused on optimizing diabetes care by adopting an interdisciplinary team approach to management, focusing on prevention and early detection, and promoting self-management and ownership of the disease. The Leader Diabetes Initiative was distinct in several ways.

INTERDISCIPLINARY TEAM

The proposal adopted a truly interdisciplinary approach to diabetes management, with a strong focus on clinical outcome measures. While the original proposal was intended to follow the ECHO model (Economic, Clinical and Humanistic Outcomes), limited time and resources led to measuring only clinical outcomes. These measures included the patient's A1C, LDL, total cholesterol ratio, and blood pressure as identified in the 2003 CDA clinical practice guidelines. Patients were cared for by, and had access to, a team of various health providers. The initiative was unique in that the Cypress Health Region contracted with a pharmacist to lead it—it was not physician-driven or controlled. True to the definition of primary health care, patients could enter the initiative through any team member.

The Leader Diabetes Initiative provided diabetes care in three settings: clinical, community, and home. In the clinic, patients attended regular medical appointments at least every 3 months. Follow-ups to lab work, medication changes, counselling, and patient education were all done out of the clinic. Although regional resources on diabetes existed, it was felt that the patients' and providers' needs would be best met by developing our own educational package. Taken directly from the 2003 CDA clinical practice guidelines, our education package focused on the disease process, treatment options, medications, lifestyle modifications, self-management/self-monitoring, clinical targets, and potential complications and their prevention.

Diabetes care and education were offered in the community through the local media, presentations to interest groups, and a diabetes-focused health fair in Leader. The health fair covered topics related to diabetes, including podiatry, optometry, dentistry, activity, and complications of diabetes. Also available were displays of healthy food choices obtainable from the local grocer, representation from the CDA, on-site blood pressure and blood sugar screening, and foot exams. This health fair not only informed the public of our initiative but, in the process, we screened over 70 local residents for diabetes.

Diabetes care in the home was primarily given by the home care RN. She played a vital role in providing education and care to those patients with diabetes that were homebound. She also reinforced teaching done at the clinic and provided the necessary follow-up for our home care clients.

SUB-FOCUS ON PREVENTION

Along with the full momentum of the Leader Diabetes Initiative came the need for outcome tracking. The clinical pharmacist updated the patient database monthly, and added new patients as they were identified. Those patients who had not reached clinical targets were identified and highlighted for follow-up, and recommendations were given.

OUTCOMES

The benefits of the Leader Diabetes Initiative were noted in three primary areas: patient, professional, and system improvements. The key improvements were noted in enhanced patient care, which came about via the increased awareness of the entire interdisciplinary team. With everyone working toward the same targets, an increase in screening for diabetes and diabetes-related complications was noted. There was also a more aggressive approach to management of the condition. As a result, more patients reached their clinical targets. The additional patient education allowed for better self-management and an increase in patient satisfaction.

For the team members there was tremendous support and team building throughout the initiative. Providers came to appreciate all members of the team and the specialized skills and knowledge that everyone brought to the table. There was enhanced problem-solving ability as all team members worked together to optimize patient outcomes. Overall, the providers experienced increased job satisfaction as the results came in monthly and improvements were noted.

It is anticipated that by preventing costly diabetic complications through the efficient use of resources that there will be less financial drain on the public health care system. Of course, the true financial effect of this type of health care delivery is not expected to reach maximum impact for several years. This initiative also promoted interdisciplinary teams in the true sense of primary health care. Patients' use of the proper resources at the correct time and place should also have a positive financial impact on the system.

The clinical outcomes focused primarily on blood pressure, LDL, and A1C results. An improvement of approximately 8% was noted in the achievement of optimal blood pressure (130/80). There was a 30% improvement in target A1C (< 7.0%), a 20% improvement in reaching LDL targets (< 2.5mmol/L), and a 15% improvement in total cholesterol:HDL ratio (< 4.0mmol/L). Although optimal prescribing was not a targeted outcome, it was also followed. There were improvements across the board for prescribing antiplatelets, ACE inhibitors/ARB, and lipid therapy.

While many improvements occurred throughout the Leader Diabetes Initiative, the most noteworthy achievement was the reduction of cardiovascular risk as defined by the pre- and post-initiative Framingham scores. When a paired t-test was performed on the pre- and post-test scores, it was determined that a statistically significant reduction in cardiovascular risk scores had occurred.

LESSONS LEARNED

Lack of financial resources is a challenge for all projects, and the LDI was no exception. It was through persistence and creativity that funding was obtained for this initiative. Funding was made possible primarily through the health region, and supplemental funding was obtained from the local community pharmacy and through unrestricted grants from pharmaceutical companies.

Continual communication between providers and establishing common goals precluded any turf wars in forming an interdisciplinary team. The providers in the Leader area are supportive of each other, and this initiative only strengthened the team environment.

Lack of timely access to providers is a struggle in any rural practice. As previously mentioned, many of our team members came out of Swift Current. Increased referrals to and utilization of these team members resulted in increased services, making accessibility less of an issue.

Reinforcing the goals of the initiative and clinical targets promoted consistency among providers. Clinical targets were communicated at the beginning of the initiative and on a regular basis throughout the following months. These targets were also reinforced through regular continuing education sessions to the providers and staff at the local hospital and nursing home.

Sustainability was an issue for the LDI. While the initiative ran from March to September 2005, it was the goal of the team that the enhanced care continue. Unfortunately, there was no further funding from the health region to sustain our program. As a result of the initiative, however, the region is working toward implementing similar programs on a regional scale. The Leader clinic is also actively involved in wave 1 of the Health Quality Council's Chronic Disease Management Collaborative in Saskatchewan (see chapter 7).

Although there will always be ways to advance patient care in chronic diseases, we believe the Leader Diabetes Initiative has provided us with a solid foundation for diabetes care and interdisciplinary team building, upon which we can only continue to build.

The Ten Commandments of the Leader Diabetes Initiative

1. Build and maintain professional relationships—it really IS who you know.
2. Recognize the contributions of each team member. Respect is imperative for team building.
3. Embrace change—don't fear it. "If we always do what we've always done, we'll always get what we've always got."
4. Work with the early adopters. There will always be someone who shares your vision. . . . The others will eventually come around.
5. Be persistent. There will be days when you want to walk away. . . . Remember, persistence DOES pay off.
6. Celebrate your successes and your failures. Columbus wasn't looking for America.
7. Share knowledge. Don't try to reinvent the wheel and don't make others do the same.
8. Communicate, communicate, communicate. It's the key to successful teams.
9. Don't try to save the world. Keep everything in perspective.
10. Put the patient first. They're the reason we're here!

11. CHRONIC DISEASE MANAGEMENT: DIABETES INTEGRATION INITIATIVE

Angela Estey, Richard Lewanczuk, and Marianne Stewart

MESH HEADINGS
Alberta
Chronic disease
Diabetes mellitus
Disease management
Medical records systems, computerized
Primary health care
Program evaluation

BACKGROUND

Addressing the diverse needs of individuals seeking health services and ensuring better access to services, especially for individuals living with a chronic disease, requires a shift from acute care interventions to more population-based service strategies. This means integration of services across the health system and better connections to primary care physicians/teams.

One of Canada's largest integrated health regions, Capital Health, in Edmonton, Alberta, provides complete health services to 1.6 million people in central and northern Alberta, including surrounding communities that extend from northern British Columbia and Saskatchewan to the Northwest Territories. The Capital Health Region's 29,000 staff and 2,400 physicians are employed across a network of 13 hospitals, 22 public health centres, and 15 clinics and community centres. An executive decision was made in 2001 to create a more effective and efficient service delivery model to anticipate the rising prevalence of diabetes and the diverse needs of people living with diabetes in our region. A comprehensive planning process was undertaken with an initial focus on redesigning diabetes specialty services to ensure not only additional capacity, but also a shift in resources and services to the community. The goal was to better support primary care providers in improving the optimal and ongoing health of individuals living with diabetes.

The result of this work is an integrated system predicated on strong relationships between clients, primary care providers, and specialty teams. The efforts have resulted in increased capacity, better access, system efficiencies, better health outcomes, and important learnings and templates for future integration of additional chronic diseases. This chapter shares these learnings and successes and briefly highlights our future plans for broader horizontal integration across other chronic diseases to better support chronic disease management in a primary care setting.

The Capital Health Region underwent system reengineering between 2001 and 2003 to improve the health and quality of life of individuals with diabetes. The result was an integrated, population-based health care system that empowers clients to take more responsibility for their health. This change was driven by many factors:

- duplication of resources between providers;
- long wait lists for diabetes specialist services, with these services available to only a small percentage of the diabetes population;
- inconsistent management of clients according to best practice;
- multiple providers and multiple service models; and
- inconsistent communication between providers, especially between specialty services and primary care.

The previous delivery system had a number of barriers to change including entrenched power structures, historical patterns of practice, public expectations, and the need to meet the constant and growing demands for services. The system was provider driven, with access to services controlled by physicians. Clients had little or no control over the management of their diabetes, and service delivery was fragmented into silos rather than organized to meet the needs of the "whole" person.

This initiative was innovative because it took a system approach to reengineering processes in a way that was inclusive and collaborative. This was not a pilot project; the direction was clear from Capital Health's senior executive team—design a comprehensive, integrated system to ensure sustainable and accessible service delivery for all individuals living with diabetes. New integrated business processes were enabled by leveraging information technology to facilitate data transfer, information sharing, decision support, and close monitoring of performance/clinical outcomes across the system.

THE PROGRAM

The new service delivery model is predicated on a strong relationship between clients and primary care providers, with coordinated support from a diabetes specialty team. The model ensures clients receive the right treatment, at the right time, in the right setting, and fosters client empowerment for optimal disease management. This approach encompasses

- the use of alternative mechanisms to identify clients earlier and connect them to appropriate services;

- implementation of a regional booking system, a single point of referral for diabetes service, and a standardized triage system with risk stratification to delegate care to the right provider;
- virtual support for primary care teams in diabetes management;
- comprehensive follow-up and 24/7 disease management support for clients;
- formal networking and access to community partners;
- ongoing evaluation and monitoring of health outcomes;
- standardized business processes regardless of where an individual seeks service or support; and
- information systems, including an electronic chart, decision support tools, and a clinical data repository.

The service delivery planning approach included development of an innovative service model and guiding principles. The Chronic Care Model (described by Hindmarsh in chapter 1) served as the theoretical foundation to ensure an emphasis on individuals supported by an appropriately organized delivery system linked with complementary community-based services. Principles guided the work and over time have become embedded in a new way of thinking. The principles focus on supporting individuals in diabetes disease management with ongoing follow-up, education, and treatment in the community whenever possible, before the need arises for more tertiary-level intervention. This means that only complex patients require specialty team intervention. There is more effective organization of care and service delivery, with a focus on building primary care capacity and leveraging community partnerships. New linkages between primary care and specialty services have been established to ensure better coordination. As a result, new roles and responsibilities have emerged for specialists. Specialists do not assume care for the patient, but instead intervene on a short-term basis when appropriate and are available to guide and coach primary care teams. The primary care teams, with the involvement of the patient, are responsible for the ongoing diabetes management. Evidence-based medicine is at the point of care ensuring a standardized, best practice approach to management regardless of who interacts with the patient.

Implementation was planned and rolled out in incremental phases. Early planning included a comprehensive assessment of the existing system, and a review of relevant evidence, which enabled planners and stakeholders to identify best practices as well as gaps and areas for improvement. This work guided implementation planning and the development of a framework for ongoing monitoring and evaluation.

ELECTRONIC RECORD

An electronic disease management system was designed to support new business processes and to ensure that data informed the planning cycle, clinical decision making, and ongoing quality improvement. The disease management system

- registers and tracks individuals diagnosed with diabetes;

- provides a longitudinal view of patient encounters, serving as an electronic medical record;
- offers recommendations and reminders at appropriate points in the care continuum, providing decision support at the point of care;
- supports workflow consistent with clinical practice guidelines; and
- allows for identification of a minimum data set and monitoring of quality indicators.

SYSTEM REDESIGN

Some provincial and local policy changes aligned well with the diabetes redesign efforts. A tripartite agreement to establish primary care networks was signed in 2003 by Alberta Health and Wellness, Alberta Medical Association, and Regional Health Authorities. These networks form a solid infrastructure to support chronic disease management at the primary care level through multidisciplinary team-based care. At the regional level, Capital Health's Board of Directors has embraced chronic disease prevention and management from both a population-based perspective and from a service provision/quality perspective. Their overall strategic road map includes individual strategies, targets, and measures for initiatives such as diabetes, obesity, and integration across all chronic disease programs. Policy changes are still required to better align financial incentives for chronic disease management and prevention delivery, especially for physicians and other allied professional groups.

One of the greatest challenges of redesign was ensuring the support and participation of key stakeholders. Principles of effective change management guided both planning and implementation with multifaceted strategies targeting multiple groups. Identifying strong executive and physician champions helped overcome initial barriers to change as the designated champions reinforced the vision and guiding principles. They were also the liaisons for Capital Health's executive team and regional medical directors' team. A regional steering committee was established as well as numerous planning and implementation teams to involve early on as many stakeholders as possible.

Redesign was done internally and was led by individuals familiar with the organizational culture. This helped to minimize risk and to address issues in a timely fashion with strategies that could be tailored to individual and group needs. A strong communication strategy ensured regular and standardized messaging throughout the organization. A monthly newsletter was widely disseminated with updates and next steps. This information was also available on an internal website.

Engaging physicians in service delivery planning was challenging for many reasons. Ongoing efforts, both formally and informally, were required to ensure their early participation and support. When implementation was imminent, some backtracking was required to maintain their support. Having a strong physician champion actively engaged in the project from the outset was critical to moving ahead with planned changes. Conducting regular physician meetings outside of usual business hours was also important since physicians were often not able to attend meetings during their clinic times. It would have been helpful to establish a physician advisory committee at the project onset, with formal links to the Project Steering Committee to encourage broader input and earlier buy-in. A physician advisory committee has since been established, and it has been well attended by members of our physician group to discuss issues and concerns and to problem solve.

Areas crucial for successful redesign included a clear organizational vision and commitment to change, a strong communication and planning strategy, dedicated planning resources, a strong physician champion, visible support from senior executives, ongoing monitoring and change when required, and an information system to support new business processes. The two key aspects were business design and information system design. Both occurred simultaneously, which was time-consuming and resource intensive. Having well-established standardized business processes and forms ahead of time might have facilitated the information system design process.

Managing stakeholder expectations of the new system required concentrated effort in the early implementation phases. Dedicated resources were necessary for this purpose, as well as a well-defined risk management plan with clear lines of communication and definition of the type of issues that needed to be given priority. Regular meetings with the executive and medical leads helped to manage issues proactively.

Triaging clients to match their need with the most appropriate service provider initially caused reactions and questions from clients and their primary care physicians, as well as the specialist group. There was a designated person to answer questions and concerns about the new system and to reinforce how to access the system. Responding to issues in a timely manner helped resolve concerns in many cases before they escalated. Historically, clients were referred to a diabetes centre to see a medical specialist and to attend a 4-day program. The new system meant that clients might not see a medical specialist; instead they were presented with service options, including group education in their own community with telephone follow-up and support from a virtual team. This was a change for everyone and required targeted communication strategies to various groups using different mediums.

OUTCOMES

A comprehensive evaluation framework was developed and used to evaluate the success of system redesign. Evaluation was embedded in daily operations, with data pulled from the electronic medical record by front-line staff. An external evaluator was contracted to oversee the evaluation process.

Success was measured by improved access to services, increased system capacity (almost tripled with no new resources), improved client and provider satisfaction, improved health outcomes, sustained behaviour change for clients, and more appropriate referrals to specialized care when required. Within 1 year of implementation, a strong business case was presented to the Capital

Health Region's senior executive, and new resources were acquired to expand the program. Another important outcome was the development of a registry of over 13,000 individuals, which represents over 25% of the total diabetes population in the region. This was a significant success as Capital Health can now effectively monitor, track, and plan for care. Currently, this registry is growing by 500 patients a month. Building on this success, in January 2007 Capital Health announced the goal of identifying and treating 100% of people with diabetes in the region by 2009.

LESSONS LEARNED

In summary, change takes time and resources. Incremental implementation steps provided opportunities to highlight small successes, which was important during our redesign journey. The dedicated team of diabetes staff who helped shape the vision and implement the required changes were instrumental in achieving the desired outcome. This team started with a small group of early adopters, and as successes became evident, quickly transformed into a more critical mass. Over time there was ownership for the change, especially among front-line staff. A few individuals did not accept change and made the decision to move on; it was important for this to happen and it was accepted as a necessary part of evolution.

In the future, lessons from this successful initiative will help guide further integration of chronic disease services in our region, not just within a specific disease, but across multiple diseases. This will enable a more seamless and patient-centred system where individuals have strong and healthy relationships with their providers and therefore are in the best position to proactively manage their health. Providers will be supported by other team members to offer optimal chronic disease management within a well-defined network of community partners.

12. THE CANADIAN HOME CARE ASSOCIATION'S NATIONAL HOME CARE AND PRIMARY HEALTH CARE PARTNERSHIP PROJECT

Marg McAlister and Nadine Henningsen

MESH HEADINGS
Alberta
Canada
Chronic disease
Diabetes mellitus
Disease management
Family practice
Health care reform
Home care services
Medical records systems, computerized
Ontario
Patient care team

BACKGROUND

Canada's health care system is clearly facing many challenges. Changes in technology, demographics, economics, human resources, and politics are only some of the forces at work. As a result, rethinking how primary health care is delivered has become a priority for many jurisdictions across the country. The National Home Care and Primary Health Care Partnership Project (also referred to as the National Partnership Project) fits within that overall context of primary health care renewal. It focused on principles of integration, coordination, and multidisciplinary cooperation. The project showed that enhancements in home care case management, chronic disease management, and collaboration/partnership—all supported by information technology—improved many aspects of primary health care including access, integration, outcomes, efficiency, provider satisfaction, and client satisfaction.

A decision was made to apply diabetes to the project model because of the incidence and rigor of research regarding this disease, and the understanding that if the model worked for diabetes, it would likely work for other chronic diseases as well. Furthermore, the clinical guidelines for diabetes (based on data from across Canada and around the world), are widely recognized and linked to outcomes. Diabetes is one of the few disease pathologies where literature exists to support the hypothesis that case management, in and of itself, is an intervention that can make an absolute change in outcomes—specifically, in improving both glycemic control and provider monitoring of glycemic control (Norris et al., 2002). A suitable reduction in A1C (a lab test that reveals average blood glucose over a period of 2 to 3 months) has been shown to decrease secondary complications in clients with diabetes, leading to improved cost-effectiveness (Ryan, Todd, Estey, Cook, & Pick, 2002). Since the project was relatively short-term, it was important to have a foundation of proven guidelines and tools on which to build.

Over the past two decades the evidence has shown that the practice of disease management and case management as two interrelated interventions improves care, health outcomes, and costs to the health care system (Norris et al., 2002). Case management is a strategy or process undertaken by *all* health care professionals (and used even by clients/patients themselves) to maximize client wellness and autonomy through advocacy, communication, education, identification of service resources, and service facilitation (Canadian Home Care Association [CHCA], 2005). The principle of case management is regarded as integral to the home care system, and "case managers" are the individuals who are primarily responsible for this activity within the home care sector. However, there has been confusion around the definition and contribution of case management within the home care context, and the full potential of case managers is not always realized.

The National Partnership Project sites—Halton and Peel, Ontario, and Calgary, Alberta—were selected based on their progressive work in primary health care, and to highlight the applicability of this project in different health care models with different home care structures and varying resources. One of the strengths of the project was its capacity to allow the unique features and priorities of each site to emerge within the context of a national initiative, thereby contributing to the richness of the project and the transferability of outcomes to other jurisdictions across Canada. There were three notable differences between the sites:

- *Different health care structures:* Alberta has a regionalized model of health care; Ontario has a centrally managed provincial health-care system, although during the life of the project Ontario initiated a transition to Local Health Integration Networks that will assume responsibility for health care planning and funding.

- *Different home care structures:* Within the home care context, case managers in Ontario and community care coordinators in Alberta have slightly different roles. Specifically, Alberta's community care coordinators provide some direct client care, whereas Ontario's case managers do not. Interestingly, over the course of the project these roles evolved and changed.

- *Different starting points:* The sites began the project at different stages. The Calgary Health Region had already started two initiatives—partnership building between home care services and family physicians, and a chronic disease management focus (the National Partnership Project benefited greatly from key findings and lessons learned from Calgary's previous experience). For Ontario, formalized, structured collaboration between case managers and family physicians is a relatively new paradigm shift from traditional relations between these two groups. On the other hand, Ontario already had a number of information technology components in place or under development before the project started.

Because Calgary clients were already involved in a partnership model of care, it was assumed that they would not perceive any dramatic changes in the way their care was delivered over the course of the National Partnership Project. Therefore, they were not part of one of the project's evaluation tools—a client survey—though it is important to note that they had been surveyed as part of the preceding Calgary initiative, and those results served as a benchmark for the project's results for Ontario clients/patients.

Other project findings for clients/patients need to be seen within this historical context as well (that is, the Calgary clients/patients had been enrolled in a chronic disease-focused, partnership-based model far longer than the newly enrolled Ontario clients/patients). It should be pointed out that the Calgary starting point also enhanced the diversity of the project with the inclusion of clients at different stages of their conditions, and providers at different stages in the development of partnerships.

THE PROJECT

The National Home Care and Primary Health Care Partnership Project was a demonstration project funded by Health Canada's Primary Health Care Transition Fund and sponsored by the Canadian Home Care Association. It was initiated in November 2003 and completed in March 2006. The project promoted integration between home care and primary care services. Specifically, the goal was to optimize collaboration between home care and family physicians by strengthening existing home care case-management roles in treating adults with diabetes. As part of the interventions, sites adopted evidence-based, preferred-practice care protocols for the defined client population and agreed on how to manage the care of persons with this chronic disease. The participants concluded that chronic disease is a community-based issue where home care can, and should, play an integral role.

The project was designed to achieve greater proactive client care with an emphasis on prevention, improved client empowerment, and more effective use of appropriate health care personnel. The goals focused on four priorities: collaboration and partnership, case management, chronic disease management, and information technology (see Figure 12.1).

Figure 12.1
National Partnership Project Priorities

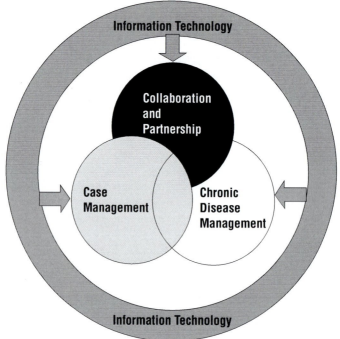

COLLABORATION AND PARTNERSHIP

In the health care context, collaborative practice refers to a multidisciplinary partnership where team members work with a client interchangeably with full knowledge of the situation and equal responsibility for the outcomes. Synergies arising from a team approach positively influence the care provided.

CASE MANAGEMENT

Home care case managers/community care coordinators are health professionals who integrate resource management and clinical knowledge, and who interact within a service network to provide information, referral, and care coordination, and (in some provinces) direct care for clients/patients. Navigation, linkage, and monitoring are elements of best practice inherent in the case management delivery model; central to this project is the understanding that home care case managers/community care coordinators have a level of advanced knowledge and practice to fulfill these roles and functions. The identification of case management as the home care strategy for this project was based on the knowledge that case management is common to all home care programs in Canada. Moreover, research suggests that a combination of management and clinical knowledge/skills most effectively meets the needs of clients/patients (in this case, with a chronic disease) in an integrated setting.

CHRONIC DISEASE MANAGEMENT

A chronic condition is an illness, functional limitation, or cognitive impairment that lasts (or is expected to last) at least 1 year, limits what a person can do, and requires ongoing care (Eochner & Blumenthal, 2003). Chronic disease management is a proactive treatment approach that seeks to support clients in the community in the management of their chronic disease and to minimize the need for acute episodic care. Although there are effective treatments for many chronic conditions, many clients/patients are receiving inadequate care. Experts report that chronic conditions are neglected because our care systems are organized to respond to acute illness and injuries. There is widespread agreement that to improve the way we care for chronic conditions requires a transformation of our health system (Delon & Sargious, 2004). Within the context of this project, disease management is essentially "case management at its finest" (Powell, 2000, p. 3). Drawing on the Chronic Care Model developed by the MacColl Institute for Healthcare Improvement in Seattle, project participants maintained that chronic disease is a community-based issue where home care can play an integral role.

INFORMATION TECHNOLOGY (IT)

IT encompasses all forms of technology used to create, store, exchange, and utilize information in its various forms. The enhancement of IT systems and approaches served to support development of all three project priorities listed above.

In Ontario, the objectives of the National Partnership Project were well aligned with provincial and local directions. The Ontario Ministry of Health and Long-Term Care had introduced new models for family physicians to work in networks or groups. The existence of a Family Health Network in Halton and Family Health Groups in Peel facilitated the establishment of partnerships with the local Community Care Access Centres (CCACs). While the Ministry's goals for primary care reform in Ontario clearly supported interdisciplinary teams and continuity of care, there was little structure in place in terms of formal home care/primary care partnerships. Making these partnerships work required a shift in the way CCACs traditionally organized their case management services. In Ontario, the project sought to move from

- home care services delivered geographically, to an arrangement that ties case management services to family doctors' practices;
- a system of centralized intake for home care services, to intake that does a better job of considering the family doctor, client, and broader health care team as partners in service planning;

- reactive or episodic interventions, to a disease management approach that is more proactive; and from
- paper-based records, to using technology to enable effective chronic disease management.

Both Halton and Peel CCACs had completed case management reengineering processes prior to the project. The CCACs were committed to ensuring that the new partnership model was well integrated with their organization-wide case management function. This meant not only addressing the need to link physician practices with specific case managers, but also ensuring efficiency in terms of geographic coverage of the regions.

Halton and Peel CCACs developed a number of tools to support communication with family physicians. Chronic disease management tools (e.g., diabetic assessment tool, diabetic flow sheet) were also put in place. The IT capacity at the Ontario site varied across physician practices with some having electronic medical records in place and others having little or no computerization. CCACs were already using common client-assessment software. A call for proposals was issued for a web-based solution to address the need for improved connectivity and automation of chronic disease management tools.

As previously stated, the Calgary Health Region had already implemented and evaluated a home care/primary care partnership model. The traditional geographic model of providing home care had been modified to link community care coordinators more closely with physician practices. Dedicated staff for partnership building, an orientation program, a compensation strategy, and a "Communication Blueprint" supported the successful implementation of this partnership model. Calgary Health Region had demonstrated that this model improved clinical outcomes for clients with diabetes. A chronic disease management initiative based on the MacColl Institute's Chronic Care Model was also underway. A diabetes flow sheet, algorithm, and other tools were already in place to support a comprehensive and consistent approach to managing diabetes. In addition, Living Well Centres had been established to provide efficient access to rehabilitation professionals and education about secondary prevention of chronic disease.

The Calgary Health Region had made significant strides in terms of case management, chronic disease management, and partnership, and this experience was very valuable to the Ontario site. What Calgary's model needed to advance to the next stage was IT to increase automation and connectivity. The National Partnership Project provided an opportunity for Calgary to enhance the three priority areas with innovative IT solutions that were integrated and aligned with the broader vision for the region. The IT interventions strove to achieve

- improved and more consistent decision making in allocation of resources,
- more frequent goal attainment by clients/patients,
- more predictable and consistent interventions, and
- proactive planning and decreased crisis intervention.

OUTCOMES

As a result of the National Partnership Project, close to 1,000 clients/patients benefited from access to a comprehensive chronic disease management approach. Although clients varied in age, the majority of them were seniors and many had a number of comorbidities. The self-reported health status of clients was higher than expected for the target population. Client satisfaction ratings were also high, particularly for their physicians, as many clients likely had long-standing relationships with them.

There was evidence of improved clinical outcomes. In Calgary, where the model had been in place longer, there was a statistically significant decrease in A1C for clients over the life of the project. This client outcome demonstrated the effectiveness of the partnership, as providers continued to achieve results despite significant IT changes to their business processes. (The Calgary site implemented two software systems, RAI-HC and Soprano, during the implementation phase of the project.) In Ontario, improvements in A1C were noted, but statistical significance was not achieved. It is our assertion that with more time for the model to mature, the improvements would increase to a statistical significance.

As Health Canada (the project sponsor) had anticipated, primary health care was enhanced through the involvement of home care, particularly for individuals with a chronic disease. Home care case managers at the project sites supported their physician partners to ensure that clients/patients with diabetes received case management interventions to assess and reassess their needs according to clinical practice guidelines and algorithms developed by the teams. Clients/patients and providers expressed increasing levels of satisfaction over the 2½ years of the project with this model of care.

Providers (community care coordinators, case managers, and physicians) reported high levels of satisfaction with the case management, chronic disease management, and collaboration aspects of the National Partnership Project. Most felt that project interventions in these areas had a positive impact on client care and interactions with other health care professionals, and also improved their knowledge, skills, and attitude in providing care to clients/patients with diabetes. Providers reported an increased level of collegial trust, communication, and information sharing.

The partnership between family physicians and home care case managers resulted in increased referrals to the home care program in Ontario. This trend was not identified in Calgary as the model had been operational for a number of years. CCAC staff in Ontario reported that the increased referrals reflected an improvement in physicians' understanding of services that can support their clients/patients. Both the case managers and physicians experienced enhanced collaboration and problem solving. In particular, physicians reported that they were able to provide options for their clients/patients, despite limited resources, due to a better understanding of the range of services available.

LESSONS LEARNED

The experience and results of the National Partnership Project strongly suggest that implementing two key strategies involving home care—specifically,
(a) aligning case managers with family physicians, and (b) expanding the role
of home care in chronic disease management—will yield significant benefits
for primary health care in Canada and, most importantly, for clients/patients.

While physicians and case managers/community care coordinators can certainly provide quality care on their own, within a chronic disease management
model, upstream care by a team of providers is considered best practice (Clarke,
Crawford, & Nash, 2002). *Quality care*, in this context, is all about clients/
patients working together with their health care team: It means ready access
to the right services when needed (with a particular emphasis on proactive
rather than episodic care), a more personal delivery of health care, increased
opportunity for clients/patients to learn more about and be more actively involved in self-care (including following protocols) and, ultimately, improved
health outcomes.

Through the project we focused on trying to understand how the home care
case manager's role would be impacted if two key strategies were implemented—partnership with a family physician, and a chronic disease
management focus. However, we discovered that when physicians and home
care case managers work in a defined structure where they are effectively
partnered, they reinforce *one another's* case management functions. Case
management on a systems level ends up being far more effective than when
these groups of professionals work independently.

It became very clear that family physicians remain the most common point
of first contact for primary health care. But the reality is that doctors simply
cannot fulfill this role alone; they require good access to community-based
services—access that can be provided through partnership with a home care
case manager. Further, by clarifying the home care case manager's role, both
members in the partnership are better able to contribute their own unique case
management skills and knowledge to effectively achieve integrated and collaborative care. Essentially, the attitude becomes supportive, the accountability
shared, and the care to the client improved.

The most notable lessons learned were the importance of partnerships between home care case managers and family physicians, and expansion of the
scope of home care in chronic disease management.

Partnership

• Reorganizing home care case managers to align/partner with family physician practices makes sense and can happen quite easily and without huge
  costs. It enables the effective leveraging of both physician and case manager skills and competencies to the clients/patients' benefit and the providers'
  satisfaction.

- To build a partnership that can achieve productive collaboration takes time. It requires the development of a trusting relationship, agreement on how best to communicate and work together, and a mutual understanding of optimal approaches to client care in order to achieve the desired outcomes (e.g., using care algorithms).
- System barriers are minimized and transitions across that system are more seamless when partners work together, understand each other's context, and strive to jointly make decisions about best utilization of limited health care resources.
- The partnership model has a broad application serving a wide range of client populations.
- Without exception, physicians who have worked in partnership with a home care case manager do not want to revert back to the traditional relationship.

Expanding the Scope of Home Care in Chronic Disease Management

- Home care has a role to play within secondary prevention and, arguably, within primary prevention. By working with physicians to proactively provide clients/patients with access to a wide range of community-based services, case managers can improve client confidence, self-care, and clinical outcomes (e.g., A1C levels may be reduced). The involvement of home care is critical for curtailing the costly crises that often arise without effective, proactive care and, more importantly, for enhancing the client/patient's quality of life.
- Health promotion and illness prevention strategies to keep clients/patients well (including strategies to prevent premature deterioration in those with chronic disease) need to be considered as equally important to illness treatment.
- Team-based care with shared accountability is more effective. Physicians can confidently delegate certain aspects of care to home care case managers, thereby ensuring best care for their clients/patients. Case management at a systems level—where all health professionals (and clients/patients) can contribute their respective skills, strengths, and perspectives—is greatly enhanced as a result.
- Focusing on system-wide health outcomes positions home care, along with other sectors within health care, to determine its contribution and accountability and to measure success in relation to a client population and the overall system.

This approach to clients/patients with chronic disease is eminently doable. To support those interested in moving forward and to ensure that the lessons learned benefit others, the Canadian Home Care Association (2006) has dedicated a section of its website to video testimonials, downloadable tools, and resources.

ACKNOWLEDGEMENTS

The Canadian Home Care Association (CHCA) is a national, not-for-profit membership organization representing over 600 organizations and individuals from publicly funded home care programs, not-for-profit and proprietary service agencies, consumers, researchers, educators, and others with an interest in home care. Through ongoing dialogue, publications, and position papers the CHCA acts as a united voice and access point for information and knowledge for home care across Canada.

The National Partnership Project was made possible by a financial contribution from the Primary Health Care Transition Fund, Health Canada. The views expressed in this chapter do not necessarily represent the official policies of Health Canada.

The National Partnership Project would not have been possible without the cooperation of countless individuals who contributed their time and resources to this exciting initiative. We are particularly grateful to those who helped to review and interpret the project findings, including site leads, site senior leaders, project partners, CHCA Board of Directors, the project advisory board, and Walters Writing Services. Please access our reports for a complete listing of project participants.

REFERENCES

Canadian Home Care Association. (2005). *Case management: A strategy for health systems integration*. Ottawa: Author.

Canadian Home Care Association. (2006). CHCA National Partnership Project, Home page. Retrieved February 24, 2006, from http://www.cdnhomecare.ca/npp/index.php

Clarke, J., Crawford, A., & Nash, D.B. (2002). Evaluation of a comprehensive diabetes disease management program: Progress in the struggle for sustained behavior change. *Disease Management, 5*(2), 77-86.

Delon, S., & Sargious, P. (2004). How the chronic care model has been operationalized in the Calgary Health Region. Paper presented at Action Centre.

Eochner, J., & Blumenthal, D. (Eds.). (2003). *Medicare in the 21st century: Building a better chronic care system*. Washington, DC: National Academy of Social Insurance.

Norris, S., Nichols, P.J., Caspersen, C.J., Glasgow, R.E., Engelgau, M.M., Jack, L., Jr. et al. (2002). The effectiveness of disease and case management for people with diabetes—A systematic review. *American Journal of Preventive Medicine, 22*(4S), 15-38.

Powell, S.K. (2000). *Advanced case management outcomes and beyond*. Philadelphia: Lippincott Williams & Wilkins.

Ryan, E.A., Todd, K.R., Estey, A., Cook, B., & Pick, M. (2002). Diabetes education evaluation: A prospective outcome study. *Canadian Journal of Diabetes, 26*, 113-119.

13. CHRONIC DISEASE PREVENTION, MANAGEMENT COLLABORATIVES AND PRIMARY HEALTH CARE IN NEWFOUNDLAND

Juanita Barrett and Ann Colbourne

MESH HEADINGS
Chronic disease
Diabetes mellitus
Disease management
Newfoundland
Patient care team
Primary health care
Rural health services

BACKGROUND

In 2000, *Healthier Together* (Department of Health and Community Services, 2000) positioned primary health care as the conduit for health and community service renewal and delivery in Newfoundland and Labrador. In late 2002, the province established the Office of Primary Health Care and a provincial Primary Health Care Advisory Committee. In the autumn of 2003, these two entities, in consultation with other stakeholders, developed a provincial primary health care framework, *Moving Forward Together: Mobilizing Primary Health Care* (Department of Health and Community Services, 2003; see Figure 13.1 for model).

Primary health care service delivery Newfoundland and Labrador includes a range and balance of services that promote health, prevent illness and injury, and diagnose and treat acute episodic and chronic illness and injury. These services support individuals, families, and communities to make the best decisions to achieve and maintain health. Service delivery planning based on needs assessments and resource availability within geographic populations (a minimum of 6,000 and a maximum of 25,000 people are served in a primary health care team area) determines the primary service spectrum in each area, thereby maintaining relevance, feasibility, and sustainability.

Figure 13.1
Newfoundland and Labrador Primary Health Care Model

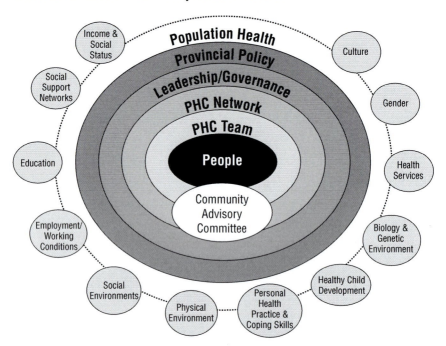

Note: PHC = primary health care. Reprinted from *Moving Forward Together: Mobilizing Primary Health Care* (p. 16), by the Newfoundland and Labrador Department of Health and Community Services, 2003, St. John's, NL: Author.

Chronic diseases, such as diabetes, depression, asthma, arthritis, renal insufficiency, and cardiovascular disease now pose the biggest threat to the health of Canadians. The prevalence of chronic disease is significant, especially in the older population. In Newfoundland and Labrador, more than 92% of the population aged 65 and older report at least one chronic disease.

With increasing obesity in our nation, we see a concurrent rise in diabetes incidence and prevalence. In epidemic proportions, diabetes is the seventh leading cause of death in Canada, and costs to the Canadian public are expected to increase from approximately $15 billion in 2000 to $8 billion by the year 2016. Newfoundland and Labrador has the highest prevalence of diabetes at 6.7%, with provincial costs projected to increase from $79.4 million to $135.4 million in the period 2000–2016 (Ohinmaa, Jacobs, Simpson, & Johnson, 2004).

In Newfoundland and Labrador, Chronic Disease Prevention and Management (CDPM) was a major focus for implementing the provincial primary health care framework, enhancing access to 24/7 interdisciplinary services, maximizing scope of practice changes, providing evidence-based services, and expanding ambulatory and community care programs to manage wait times.

THE PROGRAM

The renewed direction for primary health care promotes team-based, interprofessional service delivery. Through integrated primary health care infrastructures, publicly funded health and community services, communities, and private partnerships seek to achieve improved health outcomes, improved health status, sustainable services, and cost effectiveness. The goals of the primary health care framework are to

- enhance accessible and sustainable services,
- support comprehensive, integrated, and evidence-based services,
- promote self-reliant healthy citizens and communities, and
- enhance accountability and satisfaction of health professionals.

At the primary health care level, team members work collaboratively with clients/patients to determine the most appropriate health service providers to meet individual needs in the initial and continuing team/client/patient relationship. Within this relationship, the regional and area primary health care team infrastructure and leadership supports and enables providers to optimize their knowledge and skills. Clients/patients are empowered to manage their own health and to build healthy communities.

In the late spring of 2005, the Office of Primary Health Care, in cooperation with primary health care areas, began implementation of a new provincial approach, Chronic Disease Management Collaboratives. The provincial CDPM Collaborative Plan addresses implementation, integration, evaluation, and sustainability strategies for evidence-based chronic disease prevention and management services. The plan builds upon, and is embedded in, the primary health care framework. Primary health care collaboratives work with relevant stakeholders, including community advisory and wellness representatives, to optimize local services in support of better health.

By March 31, 2006, in partnership with one urban and seven rural primary health care collaboratives, the Office of Primary Health Care, the CDPM Working Group, and the Provincial Diabetes Strategy Advisory Committee had formulated a CDPM plan to

- implement and evaluate diabetes collaboratives in eight primary health care areas,
- initiate primary and secondary diabetes prevention activities in these areas,
- identify and engage opportunities for collaboratives in support of other chronic diseases, and
- identify a standardized provincial process for implementing CDPM collaboratives for other major chronic diseases.

Diabetes was the first chronic disease targeted by provincial CDPM collaboratives. In cooperation with the provincial Canadian Diabetes Association (CDA) network, as well as regional and local partners, primary health care teams have utilized evidence-based, clinical practice guidelines to support services to people living with diabetes in their areas. These services support the CDPM spectrum from primary and secondary prevention to management (both self-care and provider), as well as episodic interventions.

At the provincial level, the leadership team (including the Office of Primary Health Care team leader, family physician lead, internal medicine specialist, nutritionist, and CDPM program consultant) provides policy direction, change management support, and professional development. Additionally, a CDPM Working Group comprised of the provincial leadership team, team clinical representatives, provincial CDA, and provincial professional associations (e.g., medical, nursing, allied health, pharmacy, and Council for Licensed Practical Nurses) provides direction for program planning, implementation, and evaluation.

At the health authority level, executive representation supports the primary health care team leaders in planning, implementation, and evaluation. In addition, there are regional and provincial information management supports for both technology and electronic decision-making tools.

At the primary health care team level, a coordinator, facilitator, and a part-time family physician provide leadership and support to health professionals.

The major elements of the CDPM program include decision support, professional development, clinical information systems, health and delivery systems, community resources, evaluation and research, and communication.

DECISION SUPPORT

Health professionals in the collaboratives use a CDA clinical practice guideline-based diabetes flow sheet and a large number of other clinical tools to bring best practices to persons living with diabetes in their area.

EDUCATION AND PROFESSIONAL DEVELOPMENT

Provincial collaborative learning sessions provide forums on best practices and opportunities for primary health care teams to share successes and challenges in collaborative implementation. Each session is needs based and culminates in action plans pertaining to key learning in the session. Attendees at subsequent learning sessions review and revise the action plans. The first three collaborative learning sessions focused on Chronic Disease and Social Inequities, Self-Management Strategies in Chronic Disease, and Prevention. Additionally, education sessions at local levels emphasized core clinical skills in support of persons with diabetes and also highlighted the local and provincial impact of adherence to best practices for diabetes care. Provincial facilitators coached team members in clinical tool implementation, as well as scope of practice review and evolution.

CLINICAL INFORMATION SYSTEMS

The diabetes flow sheet serves also as a data analysis and service-planning tool. Clinical data is registered manually or electronically into a data analysis tool (COGNOS) that measures key indicators as well as provides information for planning future clinical programs.

HEALTH SYSTEM AND DELIVERY SYSTEM DESIGN

As interdisciplinary team members, primary health care professionals need support in strengthening relationships in specific clinical programs to best utilize available human skills and resources to provide the continuum of services—from primary prevention to episodic care. Change management processes, such as formalized team development and scope of practice changes, enhance practice evolution and service delivery.

COMMUNITY RESOURCES

Each team area has a local Community Advisory Committee, with intersectoral and community representation to direct and support primary prevention and public policy direction.

EVALUATION AND RESEARCH

Evaluation processes are in place to examine aspects of program implementation and success. Research initiatives within current processes have been elusive, especially in relationship to identifying clear methodology to test the null hypothesis.

COMMUNICATION

Key stakeholders receive ongoing communication via committees, professional associations, conferences, and ad hoc conversation regarding the CDPM collaboratives. These stakeholders inform other health providers and administrators about primary health care, the CDPM collaborative, and potential outcomes.

A number of changes are still in progress. Provincial and regional champions are actively pursuing human resource activities to sustain processes for continued team development and scope of practice evolution. Sustainable provincial and regional infrastructures to support CDPM collaboratives are being formalized. There needs to be a coalition of wellness and primary health care prevention strategies at provincial, regional, and local levels to optimize planning and implementation processes, especially at the provincial level. Early plans for CDPM data management, analysis, and reporting—with appropriate mechanisms for individuals, providers, teams, health authorities, and government—are in development, and require implementation and ongoing evaluation. Clarification of privacy/confidentiality processes, policies, and procedures for use of CDPM data is in progress, and requires formalization. The provincial Telehealth Plan implementation has commenced and will provide enhanced technological support for primary health care and CDPM activities, especially in rural, remote, and northern areas. Initial relationships among primary, secondary, and tertiary health services to facilitate optimal resource utilization have begun and will need to be strengthened. The implementation of province-wide diabetes CDPM collaboratives requires further planning; furthermore, planning for and implementation of the next CDPM collaboratives (mental health and arthritis) needs to occur.

OUTCOMES

In 2003, the eight institutional, four community, and two integrated health boards in Newfoundland and Labrador identified a number of geographic populations that would be served by primary health care teams. These geographic populations embraced a minimum of 6,000 to a maximum of 25,000 people as health service delivery populations. In the ensuing 18 months, the Office of Primary Health Care supported a comprehensive needs and service assessment, as well as a strengths and opportunities analysis process, to provide the foundation for the implementation of eight primary health care teams (seven rural and one urban) based on the provincial model. With Health Canada Primary Health Care Transition Funds, provincial, regional, and local supports have enabled these teams to change primary health care delivery based on the provincial framework and to implement CDPM Collaboratives for diabetes.

Current success emanates from cultivating champions to support required changes. Primary health care champions have provided leadership for planning, implementing, and evaluating at provincial, regional, and team area levels. Physician leadership at all three levels, including the provincial specialist for CDPM, has encouraged physician participation. Working groups have supported partner participation (e.g., professional associations, unions, primary health care team representation) to ensure awareness and buy-in at all levels. Team development and scope of practice processes have enhanced team relationships and discussions regarding shifts in scope of practice. Community development and community capacity-building processes have supported community engagement in the program, and participation in wellness activities. As well, learning sessions and provider education have enhanced learning opportunities, supported sharing of evidence-based information at local and provincial levels, and provided venues for primary health care teams to share successes and challenges.

A change environment in primary health care has been cultivated to further support the direction and sustainability of change. A population needs/services assessment completed by all teams has provided direction for change, and assistance in choosing priorities in initiating the diabetes collaborative, wellness, and other activities. Formalized, yet flexible, implementation plans have allowed primary health care teams to meet specific population needs in unique rural and geographic circumstances. Provincial, regional and local health services infrastructures have afforded interim resources to support change management, including information technology, clinical documenta-tion, and data collection processes. Physician funding model/contract development has facilitated physician participation in the planning and im-plementation of service changes. The primary health care teams have provided good information about the changes taking place to both the public and pro-viders within their areas. There are ongoing discussions regarding stability within the local primary health care core team to create an essential organiza-tional memory and expertise in managing changes and associated processes.

LESSONS LEARNED

As with any significant change, the primary health care teams and CDPM collaboratives wrestled with many challenges. These challenges were miti-gated by the activities and interventions as described above. Under different circumstances, some things might have proceeded differently.

There are a variety of things that could have provided opportunities for better success. Expanded periods of time would have allowed for better inte-gration of the changes; 18 months to 2 years provided the opportunity to initiate changes, but not to embed them into practice. Enhanced electronic health in-formation processes/systems initiated prior to implementation (for both primary health care teams and CDPM collaboratives) would have facilitated virtual communication among and within teams as well as the sharing of clinical information. Implementation of a comprehensive provincial communication strategy would have assisted with public/provider awareness of changes in primary health care, which in turn would have enhanced team activities. Dif-ferentiating, yet relating, evaluation and research in primary health care and CDPM processes would have been extremely helpful. In such a rich change environment it is imperative that we structure both evaluation and research not only to monitor what it is that we do, but also to capture its success and validity in accomplishing what we hope to achieve. Evaluation satisfies fund-ing authorities. Appropriate academic and scientific rigor in outcomes-based research can sway even the staunchest opponents. In proving an intervention successful through research, one grounds the process in the realm of "best evidence."

For the CDPM collaborative specifically, "up-front" clarity regarding pro-vincial, regional, and local implementation plans may have minimized challenges in integrating the collaborative into the "normal primary health care team practices," which would have allowed for greater sustainability. In addition, earlier formalization of the evaluation strategies for the collaborative would have clarified key outcomes and data collection processes (e.g., capture, analysis, dissemination).

SUMMARY AND CONCLUSIONS

Overall, given the short time frame of the project, which ended in the fall of 2006, the primary health care and CDPM collaborative changes in Newfoundland and Labrador have been very successful, with many changes initiated concurrently. Provincial, regional, and local direction and partnerships, in conjunction with formalized processes and tools, have provided an infrastructure for both the initial and ongoing changes. An evaluation completed in 2006 is helping to shape the present initiatives. There is significant provincial momentum and interest in primary health care and CDPM, especially in the areas where teams have been implemented. This momentum will require continued direction and support at all levels if primary health care teams and CDPM collaboratives are to complete the integration of the changes into practice. Ultimately, practice should reflect the provincial framework, *Moving Forward Together: Mobilizing Primary Health Care.*

REFERENCES

Newfoundland and Labrador. Department of Health and Community Services. (2000). *Healthier together: A strategic health plan for Newfoundland and Labrador.* Retrieved March 20, 2007, from http://www.health.gov.nl.ca/health/strategichealthplan/pdf/HealthTogetherdocument.pdf

Newfoundland and Labrador. Department of Health and Community Services. (2003). *Moving forward together: Mobilizing primary health care.* Retrieved March 20, 2007, from http://www.health.gov.nl.ca/health/publications/pdfiles/Moving%20Forward%20Together%20apple.pdf

Ohinmaa, A., Jacobs, P., Simpson, S., & Johnson, J. (2004). The projection of prevalence and cost of diabetes in Canada: 2000 to 2016. *Canadian Journal of Diabetes, 2*(2), 116-123.

14. MANAGING CHRONIC MENTAL HEALTH PROBLEMS IN PRIMARY CARE: THE HAMILTON HEALTH SERVICES ORGANIZATION MENTAL HEALTH AND NUTRITION PROGRAM

Nick Kates

MESH HEADINGS
Chronic disease
Depression
Disease management
Family practice
Ontario
Primary health care
Program evaluation
Self-care

BACKGROUND

Many mental health problems are both enduring and disabling. Two out of every five people with disabilities are disabled due to a mental illness, and six of the ten leading causes of disability are mental disorders. Mental illness accounts for 14% of lost work days, and major depression is the leading cause of years lived with disability in developed countries.

Despite the high prevalence, approximately only 50% of people with depression in primary care are diagnosed accurately. Of those who are diagnosed and started on antidepressants, less than 50% receive guideline-level pharmacotherapy, and less than 10% receive guideline-level psychotherapy. Interruptions in treatment tend to be the rule rather than exception. For example, 45% of primary care patients discontinue antidepressants in the first 4–6 weeks, but only 20% of patients are seen three times within 90 days of starting antidepressants—something that would be seen to be the minimum standard for follow-up or monitoring after initiating treatment.

Depression also often coexists with other chronic diseases. If untreated it can contribute to increased morbidity and mortality rates, poorer self-management of these conditions, and increased health care costs. Despite this knowledge, comorbid depression is not well treated. For example, only 10% of people with diabetes who are depressed receive any treatment for their depression.

The Institute for Healthcare Improvement (IHI) reported in its 2003 *Breakthrough Series* that depression had one of the best outcomes of all Chronic Disease Management (CDM) programs if implemented comprehensively, although individual interventions introduced on their own without other systemic changes (e.g., screening without access to treatment, distributing materials to consumers without accompanying education) were much less likely to have any impact on outcomes. The IHI identified four key components of successful programs:

- patient registry,
- care coordination,
- proactive follow-up, and
- diagnostic assessments.

PROGRAM DESCRIPTION

One example of a program that has been successful in making system-wide changes to incorporate a CDM approach for the management of mental health problems in primary care is the Hamilton Health Services Organization (HSO) Mental Health and Nutrition Program. The program integrates specialized mental health services into the offices of family physicians.

Established in 1994, the number of physicians and patients involved in the program has grown steadily. In 2004, the program received approximately 4,000 referrals, or 55 referrals per participating family physician—an elevenfold increase since the program started a decade earlier. The program expanded dramatically in the fall of 2005, when services were extended to all 113 family physicians in the newly established Hamilton Family Health Team. In conjunction with those physicians already in the program, a total of 148 family physicians in Hamilton have access to mental health and nutrition services in their offices. Their practices encompass almost 70% of the population of the city.

Each participating physician has a counsellor attached to his or her office (one full-time equivalent counsellor for every 7,200 patients), and receives one half-day visit from a psychiatrist each month. The counsellors are all experienced mental health clinicians who will see children as well as adults, and who are comfortable handling a broad range of problems. A program goal is for the counsellors and psychiatrists to be well-integrated within the family practice, rather than simply having an office there.

The program works on a "stepped" model where family physicians do as much as they can before involving the counsellors, who consult the psychiatrist when necessary. If the patient's problem cannot be managed in the primary care setting, the person can be referred to local mental health services.

The program emphasizes short-term care, although individuals can be seen for ongoing support depending on their needs. There are no referral criteria, other than that the family physician is requesting assistance in managing a patient's mental illness. The program works on a model whereby care is shared between the primary care and the mental health providers. All charting is done in the practices' continuing medical record—whether paper or electronic—and the family physician remains medically legally responsible for patients seen by the counsellors.

In addition to direct service, the model encourages case discussions or reviews. Educational input or advice to the family physician is often provided informally, with each case offering opportunities for brief, related teaching. Formal education sessions also occur, usually in the larger group practices.

All of these activities are coordinated by a central program management team responsible for

- setting program standards and goals,
- evaluating the program,
- allocating resources,
- resolving problems,
- providing additional education resources and materials to practices and clinicians, and
- liaising with the program's funding source, the Ontario Ministry of Health and Long-Term Care.

This team plays a crucial role in building and supporting CDM programs and creating an infrastructure within each practice to support these activities.

Over 60% of individuals referred to a progam counsellor have depression as an identified presenting problem. For almost half of these, it is the primary presenting problem. Forty percent of people seen by the psychiatrists have major depression or dysthymia as the primary diagnosis. These individuals, as well as patients with other mental illnesses, have shown substantial improvement as a result of the program. Three different outcome measures (the CES-D scale, General Health Questionnaire, and SF-8) have all indicated that between 60% and 80% of individuals (depending upon which measure is used) improve significantly during treatment.

People using the service have an over 90% satisfaction rating (using the Visit Satisfaction Questionnaire and Client Satisfaction Questionnaire). Patients are particularly satisfied with receiving care in their family physician's office, which they see as being comfortable and convenient and also reducing stigma. Providers working in the program also have a consistently high satisfaction rating. A study of community family physicians in Hamilton found that the overall level of satisfaction with mental health services was 86% for those who had this program in their office, and just 56% for those who did not.

PROGRAM APPRAISAL

For its first 10 years, the Hamilton HSO Mental Health and Nutrition Program worked effectively (an external evaluation by the Ontario Ministry of Health as part of the Primary Transition Fund demonstrated the program was meeting its objectives and delivering effective and efficient services), but when program staff started to explore the CDM literature in the fall of 2004, they realized that there were many gaps in the services. The Chronic Care Model developed by Wagner and colleagues (see chapter 1) not only allowed the program to reassess the management of specific problems, but also provided some tools to look at how the overall mental health program was functioning in managing mental health problems in primary care.

The results of this process were illuminating. Staff realized that the program had incorporated many of the procedures associated with chronic disease management—albeit in a non-systematic way—but they also identified some shortcomings in the way the program was functioning.

DELIVERY SYSTEMS DESIGN

The program had developed a comprehensive range of services. The key components that supported chronic disease management were (a) a stepped model of care, (b) the role of the mental health counsellor as a care coordinator, (c) the development of teams in many of the practices, and (d) the role of the specialist who, among other things, introduced evidence-based guidelines into primary care, demonstrated their practice, and reinforced them through case-related discussions with the family physician.

The major deficiency identified in the review was a lack of consistent follow-up of individuals treated for an episode of depression or any other mental disorder. Other than a handwritten note in the chart and a discussion with the family physician, there was no way of ensuring that treatment recommendations were being followed, that individuals were being seen at predetermined times to monitor progress, or that warning signs of a reoccurrence were identified and appropriate action taken. One other gap identified was inconsistent screening for depression.

SELF-MANAGEMENT

This was not a strength of the program. Treatment was not always goal oriented and there were rarely written treatment plans reflecting both the patient's and the therapist's goals for care. In recognizing this, the program staff identified a need to move toward (a) routine goal setting, (b) the development of shared-care plans, (c) the introduction of peer support, and (d) innovative approaches to consumer education.

INFORMATION SYSTEMS

This was a weakness of the program. The program's database was used for evaluation, but it only provided aggregate data on demographic problems and processes of care. Less than half of the practices used electronic health records, and there was very little tracking or monitoring capacity. The approach to charting was left up to individual practices, none of which were using registries. It became clear that the program needed to (a) develop registry capability, (b) be able to screen an entire population in a practice, (c) track individuals after treatment, and (d) develop routine protocols for monitoring individuals after an episode of care was completed.

DECISION SUPPORT

The administrative team had circulated guidelines for the management of depression, but it was not clear to what extent the guidelines were used, or whether the format (paper, often laminated) was the most appropriate. The guidelines were not incorporated into electronic health records, although some practices used screening instruments for depression once a problem was suspected. In addition, there was a need for greater standardization of models of care, although this was challenging with over 70 counsellors working in the program.

A strength of the program, however, was the presence of specialists—psychiatrists and mental health counsellors—who incorporated evidence-based guidelines in their treatment recommendations. These specialists received preparation from the central management team before working in primary care.

LINKS WITH THE COMMUNITY

Links with the community were also a strength of the program, largely because of the role of the central administrative team in initiating these links on behalf of all participating practices, and in providing information to practices and clinicians on changes in community activities, availability of community resources, and new programs that might be of benefit to patients of those practices.

This central team also coordinates relationships with other mental health services in Hamilton. Protocols for referrals have been developed, and the program director and manager meet regularly with representatives of all local mental health services to coordinate activities and planning, and to resolve any problems that arise.

The review recommended increased utilization of community resources and integration of community personnel within the primary care settings.

ORGANIZATIONAL SUPPORT

This was seen as a major strength of the program because of the presence of the central program team, which sets program goals, standards, and guidelines, and monitors and evaluates these activities. The program management team is also responsible for coordinating the hiring and training of mental health workers and psychiatrists, and preparing family physicians to work in the program.

In practice, the central management team has created a bottom-up infrastructure for the program—a framework within each practice for the successful integration of chronic disease management. The team also provides ongoing support through a variety of mechanisms. This model is now being used as a "platform" for the integration of other CDM programs of the Hamilton Family Health Team, such as diabetes, congestive heart failure, and obesity.

Unsurprisingly for a program with activities taking place in 65 different sites, communicating regularly with all primary care and mental health staff can be a challenge. Methods used by the management team include a website, a newsletter, email, and meetings with each professional group. The most helpful means of communication, however, has been regular visits to each of the practices. Through these visits, central program staff get to know primary care staff, monitor how the program is working, and come up with solutions to any problems that might have arisen.

KEY COMPONENTS OF THE PROGRAM

The 2004 review of how the program was functioning through a CDM lens identified several key components that were consistent with a CDM approach:

- the integration of specialists within primary care,
- the role of the counsellor as a case/care coordinator,
- a "bottom up" organizational framework that created an infrastructure to support CDM in each practice, and
- the presence of the central management team.

IMPLEMENTING A CDM PROGRAM FOR DEPRESSION

As the program moves toward the introduction of a more comprehensive CDM program for depression, the following key components will be developed and put in place:

- two screening questions for all family physicians to ask routinely when assessing someone where depression could possibly be an issue (including individuals with chronic medical conditions). A positive result will be followed up with the administration of the PHQ-9;
- protocols for care by family physicians after antidepressant treatment has been initiated;
- protocols for follow-up by counsellors and family physicians after an episode of treatment has been completed;

- greater use of the telephone for follow-up treatment;
- expanded registries to track not only individuals who have been seen, but also everybody in the practice at risk;
- goals for each individual with depression, with a copy of the goal sheet given to the patient; and
- integration of treatment for depression with the management of other chronic diseases.

KEY LESSONS LEARNED

Key lessons learned in introducing a CDM program include the following:

- Participating practices need to be involved in the planning from the outset and understand the reasons for the changes being implemented.
- It is essential to help primary care providers recognize the importance of making changes in processes of care/system organization to support specific interventions.
- There needs to be a physician leader/champion who is willing to advocate for the program.
- Counsellors and psychiatrists working in primary care need to be adequately prepared for a different style of practice.
- A longer-term change-management strategy is needed that includes regular meetings with staff of each participating practice and opportunities to review what has been happening.
- Administrative support is important in assisting practices with practical issues that arise, including space and using new technology.
- New protocols should be as simple as possible and, wherever possible, integrated with existing practices.
- Each practice needs to be able to develop its own model within central guidelines and common principles, with a clear statement of goals to be achieved.
- There is a need for a program coordinator/coordinating group to create and support an organizational infrastructure for the program and to handle problems as they arise.
- IT support, particularly for compiling registries, is very important, but changes can occur without it.
- Just changing one or two processes of care, or introducing one or two components of the model, can bring about substantial improvements in outcomes.
- It is important to integrate the management of depression with the management of other chronic conditions.

SUMMARY

Managing depression effectively in primary care is often neglected or overlooked. It requires an integrated approach that involves both counselling and medication. There are clearly limits as to what the family physician is able to do, particularly with the psychotherapies, which makes the integration of specialist resources important; however, the specialist's role, scope, and expectations need to be defined carefully.

A question for Canadian programs to consider will be whether to establish a "stand alone" CDM program for depression in primary care, or whether to treat depression according to CDM principles but as one of a number of mental health problems treated by mental health teams. Having dedicated depression-management teams will likely be a luxury; depression is usually managed by mental health clinicians responsible for a wide range of other problems. This approach has been the case with the Hamilton HSO Mental Health and Nutrition Program, which has demonstrated that introducing some components of the CDM model can significantly improve outcomes for individuals with depression and other mental disorders.

15. IMPLEMENTING A CHRONIC DISEASE MANAGEMENT PROGRAM WITHOUT TOTALLY REDESIGNING THE CURRENT SYSTEM

Sandra Delon

MESH HEADINGS
Alberta
Chronic disease
Disease management
Patient education
Primary health care
Self-care

BACKGROUND

The Calgary Health Region is one of nine health regions in Alberta. It employs over 22,000 staff and provides health care to approximately 1.2 million people. It is the largest, fully integrated health network in Canada with responsibility for acute care services, long-term care services, and public health and wellness programs. It has an annual operating budget of $1.8 billion.

One of the major problems facing the Calgary Health Region is the management of chronic illness. In Canada, chronic conditions are growing at an alarming rate. They currently affect about 45% of the population; by 2020 expect this to rise to about 60%. The care of chronic conditions consumes about 70% of the health care budget. Moreover, chronic conditions are not managed well. The World Health Organization (WHO, 2002) estimates that regardless of the chronic condition, only about 50% are managed according to clinical practice guidelines.

The solution, as has been well documented, requires a total transformation of the health system with a shift away from caring for acute illnesses and their symptoms. Key components of a system designed to provide optimal chronic care are proactive and planned care, informed and empowered patients, and cooperation among clinicians.

THE PROGRAM

Calgary's strategy for chronic disease management (CDM) is based on a "proven" model, the Chronic Care Model. The strategy builds on the strengths of our current system, as well as on previous learnings. It is intended to be relevant for multiple chronic conditions including diabetes, hypertension, dyslipidemia, chronic obstructive pulmonary disease (COPD), asthma, chronic pain, congestive heart failure, and obesity. It is designed to customize integration of the model into the workflow of family physicians' offices, without reducing clinical productivity. This chapter outlines the major components of the strategy.

EXPANDING THE ROLE OF HOME CARE NURSES (COMMUNITY CARE COORDINATORS) TO INCLUDE CDM

Care coordination and follow-up of patients with chronic conditions is being provided by Home Care community care coordinators. Community care coordinators assist family physicians in their management of patients with selected chronic conditions by providing case management, referral to appropriate services, and disease management according to clinical practice guidelines. In addition, they use care algorithms developed jointly by medical specialists, family physicians, and other health care providers to manage clients' chronic conditions.

Community care coordinators manage patients referred by family physicians either in the physicians' offices or in an accessible external facility. They spend approximately one day per month in a family physician's office supporting the management of chronically ill patients.

As community care coordinators take an active role in CDM, they receive additional education and training in the management of the specific chronic conditions they are involved with as well as in general case management. For the management of more complex/high risk patients, they coordinate specialty clinics at family physicians' offices. In addition, the coordinators link patients with appropriate community services and regional programs such as Home Care and the Living Well with a Chronic Condition Program.

In their new role, community care coordinators regularly track patients to ensure that they are following the guidelines for optimal management of their conditions (e.g., having necessary blood tests). They reinforce patients who are doing well, and follow up patients who have abnormal test results (as determined by family physicians and algorithms) by phone or face-to-face. Community care coordinators monitor the care provided using the Calgary Health Region's electronic Chronic Disease Management Information System. This system can generate lists of patients who have results outside the normal range, missed appointments, and other data.

INTEGRATING SPECIALIST EXPERTISE INTO PRIMARY CARE

Specialty clinic expertise is provided to family physicians to support them in the management of more complex and high-risk patients. Staff from specialty clinics, such as the Diabetes, Hypertension and Cholesterol Centre, and asthma/ COPD educators manage patients who need specialized care or specific testing such as spirometry. Care and role algorithms developed by family physicians and medical specialists identify patients who need this more specialized level of care. Specialty clinic patient management is provided either in the family physicians' offices or in a regional facility. Education is offered one-on-one and generally occurs in one session.

Algorithm-Driven Care

An algorithm is developed for each chronic condition being managed. The algorithm specifies the care that is to be provided and by which health care provider. Representatives from all of the provider groups involved in the patient's care for each condition develop the algorithm.

Electronic Chronic Disease Information System

A patient-centred system is being developed with separate pathways for the major chronic conditions. Currently, adult and pediatric diabetes and COPD pathways have been built. The congestive heart failure pathway is under development. The intent is to have all providers in the Calgary Health Region involved in the patients' care access the system and input data. Family physician access is also under development.

Living Well with a Chronic Condition Program

This program has three components—exercise, disease education, and self-management. It is offered in community settings such as gyms, city centres, and recreation centres. Patients can take any or all parts of the program and in any order. All components are offered at most locations. To participate in the program, patients need to have a chronic condition and be able to function in a group. The aim of the program is to provide accessible, one-stop shopping for people with a range of chronic conditions.

Exercise program: This program is run by exercise specialists with involvement from other health professionals (e.g., physiotherapists, respiratory therapists) as required. Patients with any chronic condition can refer themselves to the program, but the approval of their family physician is needed before they can begin. The Living Well staff will contact the family physician to obtain his or her approval. Patients are assessed by an exercise specialist and receive a personalized exercise program. Classes are divided into three levels (Easy Going, Get Going, and Keep Going) depending on patients' functional ability and the amount of support they need from health professionals. The program runs three times a week for about an hour over an 8-week period. On completion of the program, patients can participate in a maintenance program run either by the site or the Region. The maintenance program costs approximately $30/month. The program costs $80, but the fee is waived if a patient satisfies low income criteria.

Disease education program: Patient education sessions are run by staff from acute care clinical programs (e.g., diabetes, asthma/COPD, chronic pain, and heart failure clinics). Length of the program varies by disease. For example, diabetes education is typically a total of 8 hours and may be offered in 1 day, 2 half-days, or over 8 weeks in 1-hour classes immediately following the exercise program. Patients can refer themselves to program. Education classes on topics appropriate for people with any chronic condition are also offered, such as understanding Canada's food guide and stress management. There is no cost for the program.

Self-management program (Row Your Own Boat): Certified lay people trained by the Region lead this program, which runs for 6 weeks, 2½ hours per week. The focus is on helping patients manage their lives with the disease. Topics covered include general coping skills, taking medications, relaxation, stress management, dealing with frustration and fatigue, and learning how to talk to health professionals. Patients with any chronic condition can attend, as well as caregivers. Patients can refer themselves to the program. The $48 fee is waived if a patient satisfies low income criteria.

OUTCOMES

About 240 family physicians are working with regional staff in CDM activities. This represents about 40% of the total number of family physicians in the Calgary Health Region.

Twenty-two community care coordinators are engaged in CDM. The Living Well program is operating in 14 sites including rural areas. Both day and evening class times are provided. A multicultural version of the program is offered to two ethnic groups: Chinese and Indo-Asian populations. About 5,000 patients have participated in the program, primarily with diabetes and COPD.

The program is showing improved patient outcomes; for example

- improved blood glucose levels over time (HbA1Cs) for patients with diabetes,
- improved scores on a 6-minute walk test for patients with COPD,
- improved WOMAC (Western Ontario and McMaster Osteoarthritis Index) scores for patients with arthritis,
- decreased time required to complete a chair-stand test for patients with COPD,
- reduced weight and BMI (Body Mass Index) for patients with diabetes,
- increased confidence in self-management,

- decreased limitations in daily activities,
- fewer self-reported physician visits,
- fewer emergency department visits,
- reduced wait times for disease education for patients with diabetes, and
- more satisfied health providers.

These successes are attributed to a regionalized health system in which all components are aligned and have the same vision, senior managers who are committed to CDM and willing to try new approaches, sustainable funding, and timing. As Victor Hugo said, "Nothing is more powerful than an idea whose time has come."

LESSONS LEARNED

CHANGE MANAGEMENT

A system seeking to improve chronic illness care must be motivated and prepared for change at all levels. Senior leadership must identify care improvement as important work and translate it into clear goals and policies. These policies and goals should be addressed through the application of effective improvement strategies, including the use of incentives to encourage comprehensive system change. Calgary Health Region has promoted and implemented effective improvement strategies aimed at comprehensive system change.

INTEGRATE CDM INTO CURRENT OPERATIONS

The CDM framework has helped to guide the redesign of the Calgary Health Region into an integrated CDM management system that spans the full continuum of care. After new initiatives in CDM have begun and have had time to evolve and become more or less operational, they are moved into operations within the Calgary Health Region. The impetus for this move is to fully integrate initiatives into the regional programs, and to refine and consolidate processes and procedures. In 2006, the key components of the CDM program were integrated into the operations of the Calgary Health Region. The CDM strategy facilitates the development and expansion of the program to other chronic conditions and target groups. Both operational and strategy areas recognize that their functions are not mutually exclusive; to advance chronic care in the region, there must be close collaboration at all levels.

FLEXIBILITY: "ONE SIZE DOESN'T FIT ALL"

The CDM model can be applied to a variety of chronic illnesses, health care settings, and target populations. This allows for flexibility in services and greater opportunities to reach more patients. The Living Well Program provides a wide range of classes in different formats at different times and locations to maximize access. In addition, the Multicultural Chronic Disease Management Program offers a culturally sensitive version of the main program to Calgary's ethnically diverse populations. This ensures that cultural barriers do not hinder the access of the ethno-cultural populations to CDM services and programs.

THE RIGHT INCENTIVES FOR PROVIDERS

In order for CDM programs to make use of service providers, it is important to offer proper incentives. For example, family physicians can bill Alberta Health and Wellness for the time they spend consulting with community care coordinators about chronic disease clients. Participating recreational facilities and fitness organizations are offered the opportunity to provide a maintenance program (for which they charge a fee) after patients complete the core exercise program provided by the region. Currently, Calgary Health Region has partnerships to offer CDM programs in 15 community-based sites including rural and cultural centres.

SHOW CDM IS EFFECTIVE WITHOUT DOING RANDOMIZED CLINICAL TRIALS

Since its inception in 2004, the different components of the CDM program have been regularly evaluated. The evaluation results have provided insight into the overall effectiveness of the CDM program and have shown that the program is improving clinical outcomes, access, utilization of resources, and patient quality of life. Evaluation is ongoing, based on the recognition that the CDM program is in its early stages and that continuous evaluation is critical to its present success and future improvement. The program evaluation approach does not utilize randomized clinical trials as Calgary Health Region has adopted a "proven" model for management of chronic conditions—the Chronic Care Model—which is built on previous learning. Furthermore, our challenge is knowledge translation. What we need to do is to implement the model in Calgary Health Region's context in the way that fits into our culture and is acceptable to our patients and providers.

REFERENCE

World Health Organization (WHO). (2002). *Innovative care for chronic conditions: Building blocks for action.* Global report. Geneva: Author.

16. A NOVEL APPROACH TO CARDIOVASCULAR HEALTH BY OPTIMIZING RISK MANAGEMENT— ANCHOR

Brendan Carr, Jafna Cox, Blair O'Neill, Michael Vallis, and Claudine Szpilfogel

MESH HEADINGS
Cardiovascular diseases
Chronic disease
Disease management
Primary health care
Risk factors
Risk management

BACKGROUND

Cardiovascular disease remains the major cause of mortality in the developed world, accounting for almost 40% of all deaths in both the United States and Canada (For Healthcare Providers, Burden of Cardiovascular Disease section, n.d.). Among Canadian youth, trends over the past several decades demonstrate steep declines in healthy levels of physical activity as well as rising obesity (see Figure 16.1). Many common chronic diseases like coronary artery disease, stroke, hypertension, colon cancer, breast cancer, Type 2 diabetes, and osteoporosis share common risk factors including physical inactivity and unhealthy diet (see Table 16.1). Rising trends in unhealthy behaviours are resulting in greater disease incidence, which is contributing to a substantial and unsustainable growth in demand for specialty resources and treatment. In individuals suffering from chronic disease, the attainment of a healthy lifestyle can significantly increase quality of life as well as decrease risk of death.

There is strong evidence linking lowered risk factors among populations to improved health outcomes. Both epidemiological and community research have illustrated that the bulk of non-communicable diseases, such as cardiovascular disease, can be prevented or at least postponed (For Healthcare

Figure 16.1
Objectively Measured Physical Activity Levels of Nova Scotia Children and Youth

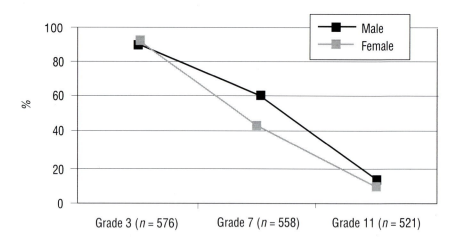

Note: Created by Campagna et al. (2001). Reprinted from "Active Kids, Healthy Kids," Nova Scotia Health Promotion presentation, n.d., p. 5.

Table 16.1
Relative Risk (RR) and Population-Attributable Fraction due to Physical Inactivity for Major Chronic Diseases

Disease	RR (and 95% CI)	Population-Attributable Fraction (%)[a]
Coronary artery disease	1.9 (1.6–2.2)	35.8
Stroke	1.4 (1.2–1.5)	19.9
Hypertension	1.4 (1.2–1.6)	19.9
Colon cancer	1.4 (1.3–1.5)	19.9
Breast cancer	1.2 (1.0–1.5)	11.0
Type 2 diabetes	1.4 (1.2–1.6)	19.9
Osteoporosis	1.6 (1.2–2.2)	27.1

Note: CI = confidence interval.

[a]Assuming a prevalence of physical inactivity of 62%. Reprinted from "The Economic Burden of Physical Activity in Canada," by P.T. Katzmarzyk, N. Gledhill, and R.J. Shepherd, 2000, *Canadian Medical Association Journal, 163,* p. 1437.

Providers, Cardiovascular Disease Prevention section, n.d.). Because primary care physicians are most often the first point of contact for individuals in need of health care, a general practice is a natural setting in which to facilitate change in patients' risk factor status and ensure more effective management of chronic conditions. Despite the evidence, the vast majority of family practices in Canada do not have the basic resources, infrastructure, or staff available to comprehensively address issues of risk in their patients. Furthermore, most fee-for-service physician funding models do not provide incentives for this activity.

THE PROGRAM

The goal of the ANCHOR (A Novel Approach to Cardiovascular Health by Optimizing Risk Management) program is to improve the risk of cardiovascular disease in a primary care adult population, with the following key objectives: (a) to improve the management of patients' global cardiovascular risk in two primary care practices, thereby improving their overall cardiac health; and (b) to increase patient compliance with lifestyle and pharmaceutical interventions aimed at decreasing global cardiovascular risk.

Launched in October 2005, ANCHOR is a 3-year $1.5 million research study underway at Duffus Health Centre in Halifax, and Sydney Family Practice Centre in Cape Breton, Nova Scotia. These primary care practices are working with patients over 30 years of age to help identify and manage risk factors associated with heart disease. The intervention, which uses a multidisciplinary team approach, is led by a physician in each primary care setting (see Figure 16.2 for key steps in the intervention). Participants are identified through a formal recruitment strategy, and undergo a validated global risk factor assessment composed of a lifestyle inventory questionnaire, anthropometric measurements, and fasting baseline blood tests. Once the individualized global risk has been computed, the study coordinator reviews the results in detail with the participant. Participants are provided with a graphic representation of their cardiac age as well as their risk of experiencing a coronary event within the next 10 years.

The behavioural intervention focuses on helping the participant to identify what modifiable factors are contributing to his or her personal risk, develop motivation for change, identify achievable goals, and implement behaviour modification. Study staff have received extensive training in behaviour-change counselling, and risk factor management strategies based on the motivational interviewing and readiness to change models. These combined strategies are applied in each individual's case in an effort to develop a personalized set of goals and strategies, which are captured in an electronic format to facilitate follow-up and measurement of achievements. In order to ensure consistency and enhance effectiveness, study staff utilize standardized scripts to guide the counselling sessions. Each session consists of the following components:

Figure 16.2
Identification and Management of Global Risk Factors Associated with Cardiovascular Disease

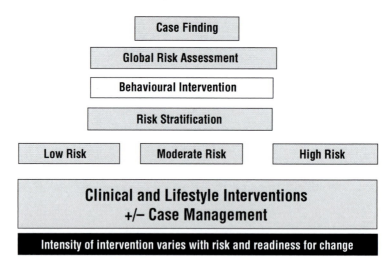

Note: From the ANCHOR program, 2007.

assessing behavioural intention, understanding the function of the behaviour (both healthy and unhealthy), promoting change, and providing a framework for conceptualizing and delivering evidence-based change interventions (see Figure 16.3).

Once the individual's risk profile has been reviewed and goal setting completed, the intervention consists of one-on-one counselling, telephone support, group education sessions, referral to other ANCHOR health care team members when appropriate (e.g., pharmacist, dietitian, exercise specialist), and facilitated access to existing community and specialty referral programs. Behaviour-change tools, print resources, and a web-based inventory with links to community programs are provided to facilitate lifestyle behavioural change (Achieving a Healthy Lifestyle section, n.d.). Medication reviews are completed and compliance is measured at each encounter for all participants. Counselling is made available to individuals who are identified as needing to start medications or when taking medications represents a significant barrier to progress. Participants diagnosed with chronic conditions through the assessment process have an expedited review by their family physician, who initiates appropriate management and referral. Participation in identified programs is tracked through attendance sheets. Global risk is recalculated at varying time intervals based on risk level.

The study is being funded by Pfizer Canada Inc. in partnership with the Nova Scotia Department of Health, the Department of Health Promotion and

Figure 16.3
ANCHOR Program Behavioural Intervention

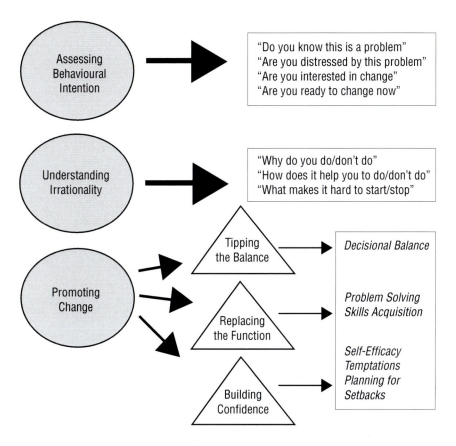

Note: Created by Dr. Michael Vallis, a principal investigator of the ANCHOR study, 2007.

Protection, the Capital District Health Authority, and the Cape Breton District Health Authority. Representatives from these groups, along with the four principal investigators, comprise a steering committee that is guiding the project. Day-to-day operations are managed by an operating committee consisting of the principal investigators, a representative of Pfizer Canada, and an external project manager. The site-based study coordinators are employees of the participating district health authorities; however, they have functional accountability to the operating committee through the project manager. Community stakeholders include a community pharmacist, physician, and nurse from each study site, and the CEO of the Heart and Stroke Foundation of Nova Scotia.

OUTCOMES

ANCHOR is a pre- and post-intervention longitudinal, prospective pilot study to evaluate the extent to which risk factors for cardiovascular disease are reduced among participating adults in two primary care settings. The research includes analysis of both quantitative and qualitative data to judge the effectiveness of the risk reduction interventions and to describe these interventions as they are implemented. The effectiveness of the approach will be examined using pre- and post-intervention measures of key outcome variables. In addition, researchers are monitoring and assessing the implementation of the interventions through process evaluation. The study includes specific measurements of baseline data, interim assessments of process measures, outcomes, and follow-up (For Healthcare Providers, Research Methodology section, n.d.).

The project involves collaboration and integration with primary health care renewal efforts and community resources to build on existing infrastructure and thereby help to facilitate sustainability. Capacity building within primary care settings and mobilization of existing resources will also help to ensure a sustainable resource. Steering committee members and other partners will ensure the project results and products are shared with their organizations and networks, as well as more widely across the province. Project findings will be disseminated throughout the province and published in appropriate peer-reviewed publications to share more broadly the lessons learned.

LESSONS LEARNED TO DATE

ENGAGING KEY STAKEHOLDERS

The ultimate success of a program such as ANCHOR lies in its ability to appropriately influence health policy and resource allocation at multiple levels. In order to ensure such influence, it was critical to engage decision makers from various jurisdictions to the point of sharing ownership for the initiative. In fact, our steering committee members have been active participants in designing the study as well as in determining key outcome variables for measurement including the model that will be used to determine economic impact. The ANCHOR model is true to Nova Scotia's vision for primary health care renewal and is seen as a provincial initiative with ownership spanning multiple health districts, industry, community agencies, and non-governmental organizations.

ENGAGING FEE-FOR-SERVICE FAMILY PRACTICES

One of the practical challenges of implementing the ANCHOR program was engaging fee-for-service family practices. Although the benefits of the ANCHOR model are readily identifiable, the costs of operating the program are not insignificant. In the ANCHOR model, the following costs are covered by the program:

- study coordinator,
- consultant resources (dietitian, physical therapy),
- Global Risk Assessment tool,
- point of care testing,
- information technology including web-based resources,
- development costs,
- handouts and materials, and
- project management.

Outstanding costs identified by the practice groups included overhead support for additional study staff, patient registration, and office space. While the dollar amount was not significant, it was critical to understand that the use of practice resources to support an initiative like ANCHOR represents an opportunity cost to the practice. In essence, the same space and resources could have been rented to another physician with the rental fees contributing to the shared overhead of the practice. Participating physicians recognized that the project would probably create practice efficiencies that would offset the costs; however, only 5 of the 10 physicians in the practice were participating in the ANCHOR project. This created an internal conflict that could have had a negative impact on the study and the practice group. These issues were dealt with by agreeing upon an all-inclusive monthly payment to offset the anticipated costs, paid from the study budget. As a result, all physicians in the practice are now participating in the study and actively referring patients.

The impact of the ANCHOR model on practice revenue was also raised by physicians as a potential drawback. In short, any model that would divert patients away from usual care could be considered to be "competing" for revenue. This issue was resolved through the understanding that the study would create several opportunities for fee-for-service physicians to interact with participants to review Global Risk Assessment scores, personal objectives and, at various points, progress on those objectives. It would also facilitate evidence-based proactive management of individuals with cardiovascular disease and diabetes, with the net effect of delivering better care through a greater number of structured visits with a team that included the physician. Because participants in the ANCHOR model would be receiving complementary services from multidisciplinary study staff, the participating physicians felt that their interactions should be less time consuming as well as more effective. These contentions will form part of the economic evaluation of the study.

SECURING SUPPORT OF SPECIALTY SERVICES

The ANCHOR model relies heavily on collaboration between community- and specialty-based resources. For our specialty colleagues, the proposed approach created several challenges. Some of the specialty services were asked to find specialists (physician, nurse, and dietitian) who could periodically come to the community-based practice to participate in shared care or education sessions. All were asked to facilitate the coordination of access to specialty programs for appropriate ANCHOR participants. ANCHOR referrals are not given precedence over other referrals in order to ensure that the outcomes reflect true system capacity and as such will be generalizeable. There has been generous support from all specialty groups for three identified reasons. First, the decentralized community-based model has been identified as a shared objective in our district health services and strategic planning exercises. As such, ANCHOR provides an opportunity for services to learn how to accomplish this objective. Second, there seems to be consensus that the ANCHOR approach should result in more appropriate specialty referrals with good community-based follow-up. Third, the model is seen as a multiplier of specialty competencies, not a driver of demand. The investment in community-based collaborative care is expected to result in knowledge transfer and enhanced capacity to manage a larger component of chronic care issues within the community-based core team.

EXPERT PROJECT MANAGEMENT

Finding qualified, experienced individuals to manage a community-applied research study was a challenge. Our initial attempt to recruit a project manager through our facilities' research services portfolio yielded candidates with experience limited to facility-based randomized control trials. As a result, we engaged a well-known local consulting firm that had worked on other initiatives including our primary health care evaluation strategy. While more expensive on a per diem basis, the overall cost has been less than a salaried project manager. The quality of the work has been excellent and the synergies that have emanated from the relationship have been substantial. Even if the ANCHOR initiative were not a formal research project, engaging an expert project manager with experience in community health models would be a critical success factor.

"CANADIANIZATION" OF GLOBAL RISK ASSESSMENT TOOL

To our knowledge, we are the first group to modify a validated Global Risk Assessment tool for Canadian use. Beyond simple conversions and conventions, our team took an in-depth look at the educational content embedded in the tool and made modifications to ensure the tool is consistent with current Canadian best practices and evidence-based guidelines.

INCORPORATION OF CANADIAN INSTITUTE FOR HEALTH
INFORMATION (CIHI) PRIMARY HEALTH CARE INDICATORS

Where possible, we have used CIHI primary health care indicators in the evaluation of the ANCHOR initiative and in the tools that have been developed to support data collection.

BEHAVIOURAL INTERVENTION

The behavioural intervention, as described earlier, is a novel concept as applied in a community family practice environment. Furthermore, the effectiveness of a standardized counselling process—which includes discrete data on predetermined indicators of motivational enhancement, behaviour modification, and emotion management—will be evaluated as a subset of this study.

INDUSTRY RELATIONSHIP

We believe that the relationship between Pfizer Canada Inc., the Nova Scotia Department of Health, the district health authorities, and the principal investigators represents a model for future successful collaboration. Not a "drug trial," ANCHOR represents a shift in focus and commitment by our industry partners to support an innovative model of care aimed at prevention and health promotion, not simply disease management. In a province like Nova Scotia, where funding to support an innovative model like ANCHOR is very difficult to obtain, the engagement of a funding partner such as Pfizer was critical. However, the company's contribution has gone well beyond the dollars committed to the project. Senior Pfizer staff have participated in all aspects of the project's development. The company has also provided specialized resources to support specific aspects of the work such as sample size estimates and health economic analysis. Our operating committee includes a senior representative from Pfizer who has been working with the principal investigators and project manager on an ongoing basis to ensure the successful initiation and outcome of the project.

APPRAISAL

It is premature to draw any conclusions from this research study. From the perspective of chronic disease management strategies, the global risk assessment model being studied in ANCHOR is an intuitive approach for primary health care settings. One of the limitations of many approaches to chronic disease is a focus on either prevention or promotion, or on a specific disease. The Global Risk Assessment approach has the flexibility to provide each individual with information and supports that are appropriate to his or her level of risk, medical conditions, and personal readiness for change. This approach also works well for persons with multiple comorbidities.

In our study, a significant amount of energy and resources were invested in creating the capacity within the primary care practice to implement a Global Risk Assessment strategy. Jurisdictions that are more advanced in their development of primary care teams, and those using office-based technology, should find the implementation of this approach much less intensive. The Global Risk

Assessment approach is complementary to self-care support strategies as well as disease management (optimization) strategies. One of the hidden benefits of this approach is that it targets common risk factors that operate across multiple chronic conditions and promotes health behaviours that benefit individuals with multiple conditions. As such, Global Risk Assessment represents a logical foundation upon which to build a comprehensive chronic disease management strategy and from which to lever self-management support.

REFERENCES

Achieving a Healthy Lifestyle section. (n.d.). Retrieved March 29, 2007, from the ANCHOR project website: http://www.anchorproject.ca/AbsPage.aspx?id=4

For Healthcare Providers, Burden of Cardiovascular Disease section. (n.d.). Retrieved March 29, 2007, from the ANCHOR project website: http://www.anchorproject.ca/AbsPage.aspx?id=1024

For Healthcare Providers, Cardiovascular Disease Prevention in Primary Settings section. (n.d.). Retrieved March 29, 2007, from the ANCHOR project website: http://www.anchorproject.ca/AbsPage.aspx?id=1024

For Healthcare Providers, Research Methodology section. (n.d.). Retrieved March 29, 2007, from the ANCHOR project website: http://www.anchorproject.ca/AbsPage.aspx?id=1024

Katzmaryzk, P.T., Gledhill, N., & Shepherd, R.J. (2000). The economic burden of physical activity in Canada. *Canadian Medical Association Journal, 163*(11), 1435-1440.

Nova Scotia Health Promotion. (n.d.). Active kids, healthy kids. Retrieved April 5, 2007, from http://www.cdha.nshealth.ca/programsandservices/obesity/presentations/NSHealthPromotion.pdf

17. A TELEHEALTH APPROACH TO THE MANAGEMENT OF CONGESTIVE HEART FAILURE

Paul Nyhof

MESH HEADINGS
Chronic disease
Disease management
Heart failure, congestive
Program evaluation
Telemedicine

BACKGROUND

The increased incidence of chronic diseases and conditions presents a huge challenge to the health care system. The management of people with chronic disease consumes a large portion of health and social care expenditures. The World Health Organization has identified that such conditions will be the leading cause of disability by 2020, and that if not successfully managed, will become the most expensive problem for the health care system. The potential negative impact of disability associated with chronic diseases on quality of life is enormous.

Congestive Heart Failure (CHF) is a health condition that occurs when the heart is unable to pump enough blood to meet the needs of the body's tissues. To function effectively, our bodies depend on the heart's pumping action to deliver oxygen and nutrient-rich blood. With CHF, the heart pump is ineffective causing the blood to "back-up" and the heart to become "congested." This congestion leads to fluid accumulation in the lungs, kidneys, and other body tissues. As a result the person may experience fatigue, shortness of breath, diminished exercise capacity, and retention of fluid (swelling). Everyday activities, such as walking, doing household chores and climbing stairs, become difficult. Although there is usually no cure, CHF can be managed by making health changes in daily life, such as accessing home support and rehabilitation, managing diet and weight, balancing rest and exercise, reducing stress, and following a regimented medication program (see Table 17.1).

Table 17.1
Congestive Heart Failure (CHF) in Canada and Manitoba

CHF in Canada
- CHF affects approximately 400,000 Canadians.
- Around 4,500 Canadians die from CHF each year.
- CHF is the most common cause of hospitalization of people over 65 years of age. Studies show that many people who have impaired cardiac function are unaware of the problem and about 30% will develop heart failure in the subsequent three years; among these, the survival rate is only 62%.
- The incidence and prevalence of CHF will continue to rise as the population ages— some estimates indicate that CHF will nearly double by 2030.
- CHF is characterized by high rates of rehospitalization, attributable in part to a lack of treatment adherence and patient knowledge.

CHF in Manitoba
- In the Winnipeg Health Region, between 1999 and 2002 around 33,000 physician visits (family physician, cardiovascular, and other) were attributable to CHF.
- Manitoba has the third-highest rate of hospitalizations for CHF in Canada with 319 per 100,000 population in 1999–2000, compared with 255.9 hospitalizations per 100,000 population on average in Canada.

Effective management of chronic disease requires a close partnership between patients and health care providers. Patients with chronic disease are inevitably responsible for their daily care, and are often best placed to gauge the severity of their symptoms and the efficacy of any treatment. As a result, they must be active participants in the treatment and adopt self-management as a lifelong task. Yet compliance with self-management regimens is often poor as a result of the complex instructions given. The challenge of self-management—which requires effective communication between patients and health care professionals, as well as access to community-based resources—highlights the need for the use of appropriate and cost-effective information and communications technology.

Telehealth incorporates a broad range of health-related activities, including patient and provider education, health services administration, and patient care. Recent literature has identified home-based disease-management programs as an evolving and important application of telehealth. These programs focus on providing care in a home or community setting with a focus on supporting the patient. There is a strong evidence base that effective disease management supports real opportunities for improvements in patient care, service quality, and reductions in costs.

The Disease Management Association of America (DMAA) defines disease management as a "system of coordinated health care interventions and communications for populations with conditions in which patient self-care efforts are significant" (DMAA, 2007, Disease Management section). Disease management

- supports the physician or practitioner/patient relationship and plan of care;
- emphasizes prevention of exacerbations and complications utilizing evidence-based practice guidelines and patient empowerment strategies; and
- evaluates clinical, humanistic, and economic outcomes on an ongoing basis with the goal of improving overall health.

The DMAA outlines six components for a comprehensive disease management program:

1. Population identification processes.
2. Evidence-based practice guidelines.
3. A collaborative practice model that includes physician and support service providers.
4. Patient self-management education (may include primary prevention, behaviour modification programs, and compliance surveillance).
5. Process and outcomes measurement, evaluation, and management.
6. Routine reporting/feedback loop including communication with patient, physician, and ancillary providers, as well as practice profiling (DMAA, 2007, Disease Management section).

The Winnipeg Regional Health Authority's (WRHA) disease management program for CHF has ensured the integration of the DMAA's six key components, which support the Region's vision of chronic disease management as a component of primary health care reform (see Table 17.2).

THE PROGRAM

The CHF Health Lines initiative began in April 2005 and is being evaluated over a 3-year period. The study is testing the effectiveness of nursing telephone support to CHF patients, using an advanced technology known as health lines or telehealth, provided in combination with the patient's primary physician. The goals of this approach to chronic disease management are to improve

- coordination and integration of health care providers to effectively manage CHF via telehealth;
- efficient usage of health care services, as evident in decreased acute care and emergency room utilization, days of hospital stays, hospitalization rates, and readmission rates;
- health status of patients; and
- acceptance of telehealth as a means of access to health services.

Table 17.2
Specific Business Rules for Telehealth and Corresponding DMAA Components

1. A patient is identified through an enrolment process (e.g., physician referral, discharge data; DMAA–1), and demographic information is reported to Health Links–Info Santé.
2. Enrolment criteria are established by the clinical team and take into account clinical indicators and the appropriateness of potential clients to manage effectively in a telehealth setting.
3. Patients are assigned to either the urban or rural group for reporting and statistical analysis purposes.
4. A detailed introduction letter is sent to identified clients explaining the program, and the nature of involvement and commitment required from participants. (DMAA–3, 4)
5. A nurse contacts the client and undertakes a comprehensive assessment using medical protocols customized for Manitoba. Through this assessment, the nurse
    *   reviews and updates the clinical profile,
    *   introduces the program using scripted guidelines,
    *   completes a survey-based assessment,
    *   collects clinical indicators,
    *   provides health education (as appropriate),
    *   reviews the proposed call schedule,
    *   undertakes goal setting with the patient, and
    *   undertakes appropriate documentation of the contact. (DMAA–2, 4)
6. The clinical decision-support software system provides for evidence-based disease stratification and establishes a systematic patient management program. (DMAA–2)
7. Correspondence is generated by the decision-support system relevant to the stratification level of the client, outlining an action plan and baseline information. This correspondence is sent to the client and his or her provider. (DMAA–3, 4)
8. Health education files, literature, and brochures are system-generated and are sent to the patient based on the initial assessment and stratification level. (DMAA–4)
9. The patient provides information to the program on clinically relevant indicators (e.g., weight gain, stress assessment, blood pressure, heart rate) derived potentially through the inclusion of telemonitoring devices. (DMAA–4, 5)
10. The software processes the provided clinical data, and evaluates data against clinical protocols. It sends a message, if appropriate, to the nurse for clinical evaluation and follow-up. (DMAA–3, 5, 6)
11. The nurse takes action based on the clinical data, the protocols, standing medical orders, or consultation with a physician or other health care provider.
12. Patients are reevaluated and restratified every 6 months using the assessment process. The monitoring program is adjusted based on the patient's stratification.
13. The software automatically creates triage reports based on every interaction, which can be shared with the patient's physician or health care provider for follow-up.
14. Patients are invited to participate in research surveys (mail and telephone) on aspects of the program (e.g., customer satisfaction, access).

The set-up of the initiative involved the acquisition of the McKesson software. The evidence-based protocol for the enrolment and treatment of CHF patients, which had been developed by the McKesson clinical team, was customized by the clinical team in Manitoba. The chronic disease management program for CHF has leveraged the existing infrastructure—physical, telephony, technology, clinical and advanced call-centre business processes—currently operated by Health Links–Info Santé—by incorporating a software enhancement to the McKesson Care Enhanced platform for the management of patients. The project was designed to compare outcomes in rural and urban settings.

A group of fee-for-service physicians in Winnipeg formed the urban component of the program. A group of family physicians in the Central Region of Manitoba affiliated with the Portage La Prairie Clinic formed the rural component. Combined, these physician groups have enrolled 106 urban and 70 rural patients from their practices. Patient enrolment was based on established criteria, with input from physicians and other service providers. The project was designed to improve integration by having physicians work with telehealth nurses to communicate about individual patient care. A clinical nurse specialist/ project manager has been appointed to oversee the project. The program set up a randomized control trial that has three treatment groups as shown in Figure 17.1.

This initiative was approached as a "building block" in the WRHA Primary Care Program's priority of developing and sustaining chronic disease management as a key component of integrated care. Linkages have been made with the WRHA's chronic disease management project and with the WRHA Home Care Program's nursing program and telehome monitoring project. These ongoing interprogram relationships are designed to align health-line strategies

Figure 17.1
Program Treatment Groups

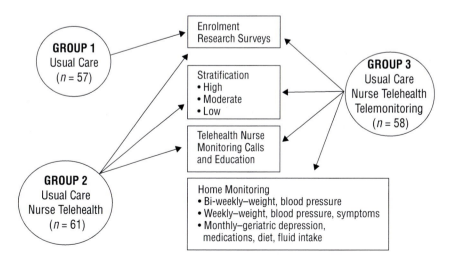

with other chronic disease management services within the region and to leverage health line support for increasing community linkages.

The approach to chronic disease management is based on the Chronic Care Model, with considerable emphasis on integration. Evidence of the effectiveness of the approach is being gathered through regular monitoring, data collection, and a robust evaluation—including a randomized control trial—of the health status of patients and health system utilization. Equal weight is given to measuring the effectiveness of integration and coordination between care providers and patients. These multiple data-collection methods will ensure the generalizability of the results to other diseases and other settings; the rigorous methods will also build in longitudinal capabilities to ensure the project's sustainability and its ongoing evolution to meet the stated objectives.

The service standards reflect the core values and objectives of the WRHA's Primary Care Program, and provide direction to staff and others to ensure the highest quality of care to individuals and, by extension, to their families. The service standards also reflect similar values and objectives of the Central Regional Health Authority's Primary Care Program, as well as Manitoba Health's principles of primary health care. These standards aim to optimize the accessibility and appropriateness of the telehealth service to patients with CHF. The initiative also drew on the Canada-wide telehealth guidelines outlined in the National Initiative for Telehealth Guidelines (National Initiative for Telehealth, 2003). In addition, the telehealth services provided by the initiative are compliant with relevant privacy legislation and ethical research guidelines, which ensure that appropriate procedures of consent and confidentiality are followed at all stages.

OUTCOMES

A number of data sources are being used to monitor this initiative. These sources include forms and surveys built into the McKesson software protocols for assessing and monitoring patients. The McKesson software has been customized to collect other data, such as patient surveys conducted over the phone with appropriate instruments for measuring health status outcomes. The software was also customized to ensure that the nurses' interactions with the clients are captured, including recommendations (e.g., see physician, go to the emergency room, self-care) and the amount and type of educational material disseminated to the client. We are also capturing data on nurse interactions with physicians and other members of the interdisciplinary team.

A content analysis of the clinical assessment and monitoring calls has been made for evaluation purposes. The Client Assessment forms administered by the telehealth nurses upon patient enrolment collected baseline demographic data that complied with Manitoba's *Personal Health Information Act* (age, sex, marital status, personal health information number, postal code). The forms also included baseline disease-specific clinical data on patients, such as weight and blood pressure, medication use, and co-morbidities. The data elements captured during the monitoring calls facilitated the analysis of progress indicators, such as changes in medications prescribed, and other changes to the baseline data.

The integration and coordination of health care providers in the CHF initiative is being measured by multiple methods, informed by the Chronic Care Model's principles of "productive interactions." Qualitative data is being collected through interviews/focus groups with provider groups and patients enrolled in the initiative, conducted in pre- and post-implementation phases. Patients' perspectives on integration and coordination are being tracked through a patient satisfaction survey to be administered at the end of the initiative. Other quantitative data gathered using an appropriate instrument, such as the Revised Heart Failure Self-Care Behaviour Scale, which has been tested for efficacy, will be vital in measuring the effectiveness of health-line support for patient self-management.

To capture the impact of the initiative on health care utilization, we are conducting a randomized clinical trial, controlling for patients and physicians. To ensure the soundness of these methods and the generalizability of the data to similar initiatives, we set up a working relationship with experienced researchers affiliated with the Manitoba Centre for Health Policy. We intend to publish the results for dissemination to other jurisdictions and internationally, to help address the deficit of research on the impact of telehealth initiatives on health services utilization.

The impact of the initiative on health services is being assessed through primary data collection consisting of patient self-reports at regular intervals during the project. We are also relying on administrative data on hospital utilization from Manitoba Health. Hospitalization and readmission rates, hospital days and days to first rehospitalization, are being matched with CHF patient data to track utilization. These indicators are also compliant with the *National Initiative for Telehealth Guidelines,* 2003. (Due to difficulties finding appropriate emergency room utilization data, these rates are being tracked through patient self-report at regular intervals.)

Health status is being tracked through a patient questionnaire (patient assessment or risk stratification survey) administered by phone at pre-intervention, and monitored on the basis of patient assessments at regular intervals throughout the initiative. The questionnaire will also be administered at post-intervention (6 months after program completion). We are using the Minnesota Living with Heart Failure Questionnaire, which has been designed to assess quality of life of CHF patients. Health status outcome indicators include self-rated health, social and role activity limitations, and health distress. Health status is also being monitored by tracking changes in health behaviour/levels of self-management through the use of well-established indicators used in assessing chronic disease self-management initiatives in other jurisdictions. Health behaviour indicators include number of minutes per week of exercise, increased practice of cognitive symptom management, and improved communication with the physician.

Improved acceptance of telehealth as a means of access to health services is being measured through patient surveys on issues such as the availability of the appropriate care at the appropriate time, with a comparative analysis of urban and rural patients. The surveys are being administered at regular intervals throughout the program to facilitate an analysis of change-over-time in perceptions of access. Based on the literature reviewed, the expected outcomes are as follows: substantial reductions in acute care resource use (hospitalizations); improved health status for CHF patients; improved integration and coordination of care; improved client self-management practices; improved patient satisfaction; and improved provider satisfaction.

LESSONS LEARNED

The program has enrolled 176 patient participants, 106 from Winnipeg and 70 from the rural Regional Health Authority. Of the 83 primary care physicians caring for these patients, 61 are from Winnipeg and 22 are rural. While detailed analysis of patient outcomes is forthcoming, some of the early results are of interest. Patients have reported many subjective clinical changes to the project staff, including increased effort tolerance, decreased edema, weight loss (68%), improved medication adherence, and improvements with co-morbid conditions such as decreased blood sugars and blood pressure measurements. Most patients (39%) maintained or improved on the New York Heart Association (NYHA) severity score, and 39% improved on their risk stratification level established at program entry.

A number of patient quotes, as gathered by program staff, are indicative of patient attitudes to the program.

"This program has saved my life."
     —90-year-old

"The program keeps me in touch with my health, keeps me more alert about symptoms and how I should respond."
     —52-year-old

"This program has given me the tools I needed to lose 60 pounds, enabling me to be able now to walk 5 miles per day. I have decreased blood sugars, which have enabled me to reduce my medications, and has normalized my cholesterol levels. I have never felt so good."
     —65-year-old

Key informant interviews have been held with policy makers, lead physicians, and other participants. The respondents were universally optimistic about the potential of this project to introduce a new model of chronic disease management in Manitoba, should the evaluations be positive. While they recognized that the project must prove to be cost-effective in order to advocate for a long-term implementation to government, there was also a strong sense of the importance of patient acceptance and improvement in quality of life. Respondents supported the collaboration between the researchers and regional health authorities. Challenges identified in building these relationships included a need for a better understanding of the priorities and agendas of each party, with neither agenda taking precedence over the other.

The need to build relationships with community-based physicians was a recurring theme. This issue seems to be particularly relevant to the Winnipeg region. Both physicians and health authority leaders pointed to limited physician involvement as a barrier. As a result, patient recruitment has proven to be the greatest challenge facing the project. The initial plan was to recruit all patient participants through their primary care physicians. While physicians seemed eager to enroll in the inititave, they did not follow through with the expected patient recruitment processes. Physicians were not expected to actively recruit their patients into the project (due to ethical concerns), but to facilitate the recruitment process. Few of the physicians who consented to participate actually met these expectations. This lapse does not appear to be related to dissatisfaction with the project processes or nursing interventions, as few of these physicians actually experienced these processes. When the initial physician-facilitated recruitment procedure failed to provide enough participants, other more direct patient recruitment procedures were initiated. Once again, physician involvement proved to be a barrier when 62 patients who volunteered to participate were unable to be enrolled due to the refusal of their primary care physicians to participate. The physician leaders in the project found the recruitment of rural aboriginal patients particularly difficult, despite efforts to involve nursing station staff in the process. The cultural acceptability of this type of program was raised as a potential barrier that will need to be explored in the future.

In terms of quantitative measurements, the early process measures (baseline and first follow-up measures of Quality of Life [SF 36], Heart Failure Self-Care, and the Minnesota Living with Heart Failure Questionnaire) did not demonstrate any differences between the control and intervention groups. This finding is not surprising at this early stage of the intervention period. It is of interest that the baseline self-care behaviour scores in this study are higher than those reported in literature from the United States. The maximum attainable score on this measure is 145, and the literature reports scores in the range of 86 with a standard deviation of 30. The baseline functional level of participants in the study was higher with an average score of 130. This high level of self-care at the onset of the study leaves less opportunity for improvement.

We are taking steps to ensure the sustainability of this project, with the overarching view of the initiative as a "building block" for larger changes on a number of levels of care. The execution of a robust evaluation, based in part on a randomized control trial, will ensure the generalizability of the results to similar initiatives for other chronic diseases or different patient and provider populations. We are also building on work being done in other areas to improve our processes and linkages. We are working closely with the WRHA

ABC Project on chronic disease management to decrease admissions in the acute care sector, as well as with the Home Care Program's telehome monitoring program to incorporate aspects of the home care nursing program into the team approach to CHF management.

REFERENCES

Disease Management Association of America (DMAA). (2007). Disease Management section. Retrieved April 10, 2007, from the DMAA website, http://www.dmaa.org/dm_definition.asp

National Initiative for Telehealth. (2003). *National Initiative for Telehealth Guidelines*. Ottawa: Framework of Guidelines.

SYNTHESIS AND CONCLUSION

18. SYNTHESIS OF REPORT-BACK SESSION AT THE NATIONAL CHRONIC DISEASE MANAGEMENT CONFERENCE APRIL 6–7, 2006, TORONTO

Michael Hindmarsh and Nick Kates

INTRODUCTION

This working conference brought together over 110 Chronic Disease Management (CDM) leaders in the field, key stakeholders, and federal/provincial/territorial jurisdiction representatives to share experiences, lessons learned, and next steps in implementing successful CDM initiatives in primary health care. There were five plenary presentations showcasing flagship programs in Canada, the United States and the United Kingdom, and 20 breakout sessions on innovative CDM initiatives in primary health care representing almost all jurisdictions in Canada. This chapter offers a summary of the recommendations that arose out of the final plenary session.

The Wagner Chronic Care Model is the basis for most of the activity currently underway in Canada in chronic disease management. Several jurisdictions have adapted it to incorporate a broader view of community and to emphasize prevention and population health. The Wagner model is a disease-neutral approach; however, many of its applications refer to specific diagnostic groups. It is important to look at how CDM programs for different diseases can be integrated, preferably from the planning stage forward. There is much overlap between chronic diseases in both risk factors and strategies for improvement. At the same time, there also needs to be enough flexibility to incorporate disease-specific approaches into this framework. Initiatives should be considered that reach the largest number of Canadians. Using an integrated approach to multiple problems, it is possible to address common risk factors for primary and secondary prevention.

There were numerous subthemes throughout the conference. Organizing them by the components of the Chronic Care Model is a useful way to summarize these themes. All the components of the model are interrelated and need to be considered when building a CDM program.

INFORMATION TECHNOLOGY (IT)

IT is critical infrastructure to enable efficient, effective, integrated, comprehensive, and continuous population-based care. IT supports communication, information transfer and exchange, decision making, performance measurement, and process and outcome evaluation. Comprehensive and standardized IT strategies need to be developed at the provincial (if not at the national) level. Disparate IT systems scattered across catchment areas will only lend more chaos to the current situation.

COMMUNITY LINKAGES

Care navigation, clinical case management, and integration across services are key. The notion of primary care being the medical home that other systems coordinate with is being considered in other countries. Partnership development and relationship building are needed to support sustainable programs. Linkages with social services, as well as with community mental health services, must be fostered and expanded.

PATIENT SELF-MANAGEMENT

Self-management needs to be seen as a central component of CDM. Training for primary practice teams to deliver self-management support at every encounter and to build self-management programs in the community must be a priority in future work. Programs are needed to teach patients self-care as well as appropriate use of health care services. Self-management services must be organized around patient needs, with care following the patient instead of residing in multiple providers' offices.

PRACTICE REDESIGN

Practice redesign should support new roles for primary health care providers by building infrastructure. The team approach extends beyond primary care to include specialists, home care, long-term care, and inpatient care. Flexible models are needed to allow for adaptation to local contexts, cultural differences, community needs and resources. Alternatives to the individual office visit may be needed, such as the use of group visits, and telephone or email visits and follow-ups.

DECISION SUPPORT AND TRAINING

It is essential to build and leverage the capacity of primary health care providers, specialists, community services, and lay people to use IT for effective care delivery, performance measurement, and evaluation. It is also desirable to support links between practice settings and academic institutions and to establish a repository of best CDM practices.

HEALTH CARE ORGANIZATION

Strategies to change care-delivery patterns may include incentives to provide quality chronic care—incentives that recognize the different delivery models needed to care for these patients. It may make sense to increase reimbursement for group visits, telephone follow-up, and planned chronic care encounters. It is essential to align incentives with expected outcomes in order to build the business case for investing in CDM in primary health care.

IMPLEMENTATION APPROACHES

Summarized below are suggestions that emerged throughout the session. While not inclusive of all ideas put forth, they do represent those that had general agreement in the audience.

- CDM programs should be implemented with a long-term perspective. Patience is called for, as well as sensitivity to the culture of primary care, the population being served, and differences between rural and urban, small and large practices. However, planning should not be a protracted process. Moving quickly and testing implementation ideas on a small scale will inform the process better than large-scale planning.
- There needs to be identified physician "champions" and strong local leaders for these programs to work. Similarly, there must be committed leadership at the regional and provincial levels. Grassroots efforts, no matter how successful, will languish without broader system support.
- Successful programs appear to have begun by focusing on the early adopters. Successful adopters can function as change agents for others.
- There is a need for funding if these programs are to work. Providers cannot be asked to work harder or to squeeze improvement in during their lunch hour. Quality improvement infrastructure must be built to support change at the practice level. For example, the Local Health Integration Networks in Ontario could serve as "Centres for Excellence" whose mission is to support system change among Family Health Teams.
- Preparation of providers is essential. Training collaboratives, based upon models developed by the MacColl Institute and the Institute for Healthcare Improvement, seem to be the most effective way of changing provider behaviour. Follow-up and peer support seem to be important components of the success of these models. There should be a comprehensive review of what works and doesn't work vis-à-vis quality improvement.
- Marketing to consumers and providers is an important part of the implementation of these programs.
- CDM approaches need to be built, wherever possible, upon existing protocols within practices. It will also be useful to examine practice function to determine where duplication can be eliminated.
- The creation of a National Clearinghouse for implementation strategies, tools, and so forth should be established based on the best practices from Canada and internationally.
- Forums for the ongoing sharing of best practices and other learnings should be a priority.

- Create environments to support innovation, risk taking, and ongoing change—a culture of improvement.
- Support improved evaluation and data collection at different levels (system, provider, patient). There cannot be knowledge of improvement without good data.

19. CONCLUSION AND DIRECTIONS FOR THE FUTURE

Mary Ann McColl and John Dorland

We began this book by emphasizing the size and scope of the challenge that is before health care systems in Canada to respond to the growing threat of chronic disease. Based on the assumption that existing structures aimed at acute care cannot effectively and efficiently meet this challenge, a recent focus has been on Chronic Disease Management (CDM) in primary health care. As stated, this book grew out of a national invitational conference on CDM featuring leaders in this emerging field in Canada, as well as recognized experts from the United States and the United Kingdom. The previous chapter offered a synthesis of the conference, derived from the closing plenary and the deliberations of the various breakout groups. The aim of the book is to bring the results of that conference to a wider audience and to contribute to the national and international debate about chronic disease management. To that end, we have the privilege of offering some concluding thoughts arising out of the collected contributions of these committed individuals.

THEORETICAL UNDERPINNINGS

Three theoretical tools have emerged that appear to have provided shape and substance to the leading programs internationally and here in Canada. These models are, first and foremost, the Chronic Care Model, originally developed by Wagner and colleagues from the Group Health Collaborative in Seattle, Washington, and subsequently adapted for its first Canadian application in British Columbia (see chapter 3); second, the Kaiser Permanante Risk Pyramid; and third, the Institute for Healthcare Improvement's learning collaborative process.

THE CHRONIC CARE MODEL

Since its inception less than a decade earlier, the Chronic Care Model has become the *lingua franca* of chronic disease management, and is cited by almost every program reviewed in this volume as the basis for its design and structure. The Chronic Care Model provides a way of thinking about essential elements of chronic disease management that need to be assembled in order to begin contemplating the development of a program. The model identifies six elements, including a community that is receptive to linkages with primary care and that offers the necessary services. Using this model, proponents can assess the readiness of their practice to embark on a CDM program, and begin to assemble the human and material resources needed to move ahead.

THE KAISER RISK PYRAMID

Another interesting observation pertaining to the preceding chapters is the utility of the Kaiser Risk Pyramid in focusing the attention of primary care providers on the subset of a typical caseload that is most in need of chronic disease management. The Risk Pyramid, described in detail in chapter 2, partitions patients of a primary care practice into three groups: those who can effectively be served by the family doctor alone (about 60 to 80%); those who need "care management"—that is, additional support to engage in effective self-management (about 20%); and finally, the small percentage (estimated at 5 to 6%) who have multiple or complex chronic conditions that require more from primary health care than the conventional family practice can deliver. Although this latter group represents a small contingent within the practice, they are inordinately high consumers of service. Their needs include both medical and social issues, which have been shown to be most effectively addressed in a multidisciplinary environment, coordinated by a case manager.

Unlike the Chronic Care Model, the Risk Pyramid has not been widely quoted by the various chapter authors. Despite the fact that it too derives from a key American pioneer in the field of chronic disease management, the Risk Pyramid has not pervaded the consciousness of providers in the same way that the Chronic Care Model has done. This apparent oversight may simply be a consequence of the manner of dissemination of these two theoretical tools; however, the Risk Pyramid is a highly useful way of thinking about a number of aspects of practice design and management, from resource allocation to documentation. It assists in the identification of high risk individuals, thus delimiting the scope of concern for CDM programs. It allows practitioners to draw boundaries around those patients who will be targeted for case management and more intensive service, and to develop disease and demographic profiles for that group. For a good example of how the Kaiser Risk Pyramid may be used for resource and service planning, see Rosen's chapter detailing the very deliberate and systematic design of the English CDM program.

INSTITUTE FOR HEALTHCARE IMPROVEMENT'S COLLABORATIVE PROCESS

Both the Chronic Care Model and the Kaiser Risk Pyramid offer useful theoretical bases for the design of CDM programs. After design comes implementation, and this requires a third type of knowledge to institute necessary changes to historical systems and participants' behaviour. This essential step in successful implementation is often underestimated. Proven theoretical bases for this aspect of the endeavour are harder to come by. A method that several programs found to be effective was the U.S. Institute for Healthcare

Improvement's "collaboratives" process. Learning collaboratives were fundamental to the English CDM transformation, described by Rosen, and to the excellent British Columbia program described by Macgregor. The Saskatchewan program also used the collaborative process as the basis for its implementation stage. Chan's chapter provides a good description of the Saskatchewan program and of the application of the Institute for Healthcare Improvement's collaborative process.

DISEASE-SPECIFIC PROGRAMS

Many of the programs reviewed began with single-disease models of CDM, with the intention of moving to more generic models in the future. Furthermore, the single diseases chosen are highly predictable. A review of the keywords associated with the chapters reveals that most often diabetes, heart disease, hypertension, and mental illness are the focus of chronic disease management. These conditions have important public health implications. Perhaps more importantly, these conditions tend to have well-developed clinical guidelines for practice and an acceptable range of treatment options. This specific-to-general direction of program development appears to have occurred in many jurisdictions, despite continuing appeals in the literature to adopt a generic approach to chronic disease management. Arguably, once the technology and human resources are in place to practise CDM with respect to one condition, the transition to either an additional condition or a more generic model becomes much easier.

INFORMATION TECHNOLOGY INFRASTRUCTURE REQUIREMENT

One point that comes through strongly in all of the papers is the need for a solid information technology (IT) infrastructure. In many other sectors of the health care system, the introduction of IT support improves efficiency and patient care. In chronic disease management, however, it is an integral part of the program, and is thus essential. CDM programs simply cannot be implemented without the appropriate integrated IT components. This requirement derives from the inherent nature of a typical CDM program, which involves identifying and classifying patients, continual accumulation of clinical data from various sources, timely sharing of patient information among many health/ community service providers, and long-term tracking of patient progress.

A second point regarding IT is that this infrastructure needs to be an integral part of the larger health care system. It is neither practical nor cost effective in the long-term for CDM programs to build their own systems, at least for fundamental functions such as patient rosters, electronic clinical records, and interagency data communication.

The corollary to this is that the lack of an existing comprehensive, integrated IT infrastructure in the broader health care system would create a major hindrance to the development and proliferation of effective CDM programs. Unfortunately, this may be the situation in many Canadian jurisdictions.

HISTORICAL CONTEXT

An interesting observation is the number of programs described in this book that experienced a "bottom-up" rather than a "top-down" process of development. Take for example the Group Health Centre in Sault Ste. Marie, Ontario (chapter 4). Crookston and Bodnar briefly summarize the dramatic history of community involvement and grassroots participation that led to the successful development of their program. Chapter 10 provides another example of community initiative as the engine for program development. In this case, Millar describes the efforts of a local pharmacist who identified the need for improved diabetic care, and acted as the catalyst for change. These and other examples of community participation in CDM programs highlight the relatively small proportion of elements of the Chronic Care Model that pertain specifically to the practice itself, and the many other elements that need to come from the community in order for a program to succeed. Sustainability has been identified by a number of programs as an issue, particularly for those that began as a result of research grants or Primary Health Care Transition Fund projects. To the extent that the community is involved in the program, and especially if the community has an investment of energy and commitment to the program, the chances increase that the resources needed for sustainability will be secured.

PHYSICIAN LEADERSHIP VS. MULTIDISCIPLINARY TEAM PERFORMANCE

A further observation from the preceding chapters is the juxtaposition of recommendations about the need for physician leadership and the need for effective team functioning. Some readers may feel that these two recommendations are in opposition to one another—that in order for effective team functioning to occur, there can be no implicit or explicit hierarchy within the team, particularly if one discipline (medicine) is identified as the de facto leader in all cases.

In most jurisdictions in Canada, primary health care is funded on the basis of physician workload units. Other than in salaried models of funding, which are admittedly in the minority, primary health care organizations receive revenues on the basis of the number of work units generated by the physicians (fee-for-service) or the number of patients rostered to the physicians (capitation). Thus the funding structure places physicians in a different relationship to the team than other service providers, such as allied health professionals. Strictly speaking, non-physician members of the team are dependent upon physicians for generating the revenues needed to operate the practice. As long as this is the case (and there is no evidence that this funding structure will change in the foreseeable future), then it is clear that the team will not be constituted of "equals" in the eyes of the organization or the payers.

This organizational reality need not stand in the way of effective multidisciplinary team functioning; however, it will require the development of mature interdisciplinary relationships based on mutual respect and appreciation for the contributions of each team member. While allied health professionals are typically trained to function in an interdisciplinary team, this is not always the case for physicians. Physicians are trained and professionally socialized to take ultimate responsibility for patients. Furthermore, they are legally responsible and professionally liable for patients in their care. Such circumstances are not conducive to joint management or shared authority for patient care. Thus we have a potential clash of expectations with regard to how clinical decisions are made and how accountabilities are enacted. While physicians expect to bear responsibility and authority, other health professionals expect to share in that responsibility.

Further, the literature suggests that family physicians are particularly disposed toward a high degree of independence in their mode of practice. In many cases, it is this very independence, autonomy, and sole responsibility that attracted them to family practice, rather than to one of the other medical specialties that tends to be practiced within the context of a larger organization or institution. Thus for family physicians, team functioning may be an even more uncommon and perhaps even uncomfortable fit than it is for specialists, who more frequently work side by side with other professionals.

The preceding chapters on successful CDM programs have offered relatively little discussion of this complex issue, other than to observe that both physician leadership and effective team functioning are necessary for good chronic disease management. This is a sensitive issue that involves professional role definitions and boundaries, joint accountabilities, personal egos, and interprofessional respect. As CDM programs evolve to include the broader array of professionals needed to serve the needs of people with multiple chronic conditions, this is an issue to be tracked and evaluated. Important lessons learned from successful programs then need to be incorporated into the professional training and continuing education of both medical and allied health professionals. There is evidence that when students in different professions are trained together, they learn to function together effectively and respectfully. And yet interdisciplinary education in the health professions is still more the exception than the norm. Chronic disease management is a growing area of health care that may act as a catalyst for this long overdue development in the education of future health professionals.

POLICY ALIGNMENT

Another crucial factor in successful implementation of CDM programs is proper alignment of overall health-system policies with the goals and requirements of chronic disease management. There is no chance for a new program to flourish, however expertly and enthusiastically championed, if the underlying policy structure and its inherent economic incentives are pushing in another direction. This theme is emphasized in Rosen's chapter on the English experience. It is also brought out, indirectly, in the chapter on the Group Health Centre (GHC) in Sault Ste. Marie, Ontario, contributed by Crookston and Bodnar. When it originated several decades ago, the GHC was an innovative, locally sponsored program. However, for years many of its innovative features, including non-fee-for-service funding, integrated health programs, and community boards, did not align with provincial health policies. As a result, the GHC was engaged in continual struggle for funding, support and recognition. Recently, however, provincial health policies, particularly those relating to primary health care, have shifted to more closely align with the GHC features. As a result, the GHC now finds itself it a much more comfortable situation, and was accorded a featured place in the plenary session at the April 2006 conference.

Is the Canadian health policy structure well-aligned with CDM goals and requirements? *Well*-aligned might be too strong, but policies do seem to be moving in the right direction. The main policy elements needed to support CDM programs are funding structures that encourage seeking out patients with chronic conditions; delegation of services to the appropriate health or community provider; continual monitoring without unnecessary intervention; and regulatory, educational, and other structures that encourage interdisciplinary teamwork. The policy reforms in primary health care taking place across Canada, although variable and incomplete, are very promising, and should provide a fertile policy structure for chronic disease management. Policies promoting interdisciplinary teamwork, as discussed above, still appear to have some distance to go.

COST-EFFECTIVENESS AND SUSTAINABILITY

Many of the programs discussed in this book are at an early stage of development, and do not yet have a long history of outcomes. Even those that do have measured outcomes did not relate them to costs (at least not in these papers). Furthermore, since many programs are relatively new, and perhaps even running in a pilot mode, current costs will not provide a fair estimate of the costs of a stable, long-term program.

Nevertheless, whether these programs are cost-effective and sustainable will be the next pressing question, after successful outcomes are demonstrated. The work to determine financial viability must be done if these CDM programs are to flourish countrywide, and become an integral part of the Canadian health system.

At this point, all we can offer is grounded optimism. Chronic disease management has many characteristics that promise cost-effectiveness. Firstly, the programs are largely low-tech: unlike many health innovations, they do not require expensive new technology. They use services, technology, and health personnel that already exist—the new requirement is reorganization. Secondly, they incorporate a large component of self-management which, aside from the training and support effort, does not entail more health system costs. Also, the self-management aspect incorporates a strong preventive element which, if successful, will reduce future acute care needs. Thirdly, the programs appear to produce results. Those that have been running long enough to track outcomes are demonstrating some remarkable results. See, for example, the chapter by Macgregor on the British Columbia CDM program, and by Crookston and Bodnar on the Group Health Centre in Ontario.

Thus, both the early outcomes and the underlying cost structure of CDM programs hold promise for a good cost-effectiveness story. We hope that this will be confirmed when definitive results become available.

CONCLUSION AND RECOMMENDATIONS

In summary, this book draws on the knowledge of international and national leaders in CDM in primary health care. Its aim is to advance the debate about chronic disease management by taking a pulse on this emerging field, and summarizing lessons learned at this critical juncture in Canadian health care. The preceding chapter highlighted the findings of the invitational conference that gave rise to the book, and the foregoing discussion attempted to summarize themes and issues emerging out of the experiences of these pioneers. Several recommendations conclude our discussions and hopefully will spark debate and action.

1. Given the widespread adoption of the three theoretical tools described above (the Chronic Care Model and, to a lesser but significant extent, the Kaiser Risk Pyramid and the Institute for Healthcare Improvement's collaborative process), we recommend that individuals proposing or contemplating new programs take advantage of the assistance offered by these tools. Further model development appears unwarranted, except in the most unusual of contextual circumstances. Even extensive adaptation of these theoretical tools must be clearly justified, given the broad base of support that exists in the field for these approaches. This is not to say that the field should become monolithic or exclusive, because new ways of thinking are always welcome. However, it does suggest that there are reasonable tools already available to assist practitioners to develop new programs without the necessity of starting from scratch. The Chronic Care Model can assist in assessing the availability and degree of development of the six model elements, the Kaiser Risk Pyramid can assist in identifying the subset of the caseload to be the focus of initial efforts, and learning collaboratives can assist in creating an environment that is compatible with change. The development and implementation of new programs should not be delayed due to a perceived need for a theoretical framework.

2. A second recommendation arising out of the preceding chapters is to re-
    sist the temptation to focus exclusively on single diagnosis programs, and
    instead to begin to develop broad spectrum CDM programs. One way of
    approaching this task is to focus on risk factors rather than on the dis-
    eases they are associated with. For example, a program might focus on
    obesity (waist circumference), a risk factor about which current research
    offers considerable guidance. This approach would not only capture many
    of the major diagnostic groups that are currently the focus of CDM pro-
    grams, but would also offer the opportunity to become involved with
    primary and secondary prevention as well as chronic disease manage-
    ment. Primary prevention focuses on the whole population, attempting to
    prevent the risk of disease. Secondary prevention focuses on those al-
    ready at risk, attempting to prevent the onset of disease. Tertiary prevention
    focuses on those already diagnosed with a particular disease, and attempts
    to prevent them from developing complications, secondary diagnoses, and
    disabilities. Some authors also identify a fourth level of prevention, aimed
    at those who already have complicated conditions. Quaternary preven-
    tion attempts to prevent this complex subset of the population from
    becoming socially disadvantaged and entering a spiral of illness, poverty,
    and isolation. It is between these latter two categories of prevention that
    disease-specific CDM programs currently sit.
3. A third recommendation that appears to issue from these model programs
    is the need for central leadership, particularly in two areas: policy and
    information technology. It has been shown in a number of the programs
    that the presence of aligned policy and appropriate economic incentives
    lead to an environment that supports and encourages programming inno-
    vation, rather than locking professionals into practice patterns that fail to
    respond to the needs of the population. While governments are under-
    standably reluctant to govern the practice environment too closely, there
    are considerable efficiencies to be realized by offering leadership on tech-
    nical issues like information technology. In order to facilitate change in a
    massive sector like the health care system, where vested interests and
    role boundaries often stand in the way, governments with a clear policy
    direction and a bold implementation plan are needed to effect significant
    improvements.
4. A fourth recommendation that derives from the preceding chapters is a
    recognition of the role that communities can play in initiating and sus-
    taining chronic disease management. Community initiatives brought
    several of the programs into reality, while at the same time ensuring the
    relevance of program elements to the particular needs of the population.
    Regional governments may also play a role in integrating and coordinat-
    ing the many community components needed to make a success of chronic
    disease management. Communities should be broadly defined to include
    both geographic communities, and communities of affiliation such as con-
    sumer advocacy groups and voluntary organizations.

5. The need for interdisciplinary teams in order to do CDM in primary health care gives rise to a fifth recommendation. Despite decades of discussion of the benefits of interdisciplinary health care, it is still the reality only in small pockets of the health care system. The research clearly shows that if professionals are expected to work together, they must be educated together. They must learn about each other's roles not in a one-hour lecture or inservice, but through sustained contact and the development of working relationships and interprofessional trust. Often logistical difficulties stand in the way of interdisciplinary professional education and practice, despite the best of intentions. Post-secondary educational institutions need to be brought into the debate about chronic disease management so that they are adequately preparing new professionals for roles in these programs. Further, existing CDM programs need support to overcome the challenges of interprofessional practice. It cannot be assumed that goodwill alone will effect this transition. Chronic disease management programs need to be specifically resourced to permit regular team meetings, as well as occasional team development sessions.

6. Finally, many of the authors contributing chapters to this book indicate that they are involved in a process of focused program evaluation, with the intention of presenting and publishing their findings. This book and the 2006 conference have provided an opportunity for program leaders to assemble their thoughts and share their experiences. If chronic disease management is to continue to progress as it has in recent years, the extraordinary efforts of these pioneers will have to be repeated in practices across the country. Much of this development, both clinical and intellectual, has been fuelled by the opportunity created by the Primary Health Care Transition Fund. New sources of funding will bring renewed energy for discovery, development, and dissemination of findings as the field of chronic disease management goes forward.

APPENDIX
CONTRIBUTORS TO THE CONFERENCE ORGANIZATION

The chapters in this book are based on presentations made at the National Chronic Disease Management Conference (CDM) held in Toronto, Canada, on April 6–7, 2006. Thanks are due to many people and organizations for their contributions to the planning and implementation of the conference:

- The National CDM Conference Steering Committee members
  - Louise Rosborough, Manager (Acting), Primary and Continuing Health Care Division, Health Canada
  - Georgina Georgilopoulos, Policy Analyst, Primary and Continuing Health Care Division, Health Canada
  - Dr. Gregory Taylor, Director General, Centre for Chronic Disease Prevention and Control, Public Health Agency of Canada
  - Dr. Chris Rauscher, Chair, Province-wide Chronic Disease Collaborative for Patients with Congestive Heart Failure in British Columbia
  - Dr. Howard Platt, Former Director, Medical Outcomes Improvement Branch, British Columbia Ministry of Health Services
  - Juanita Barrett, Team Leader, Office of Primary Health Care, Newfoundland Department of Health and Community Services
  - Dr. Ann Colbourne, Associate Professor, Department of Medicine, Memorial University of Newfoundland
  - Dr. Nick Kates, Program Director, Hamilton Family Health Team, Ontario
  - Susan Sue-Chan, Director (Acting), Finance, Accountability and Information, Primary Health Care and Family Health Teams, Ontario Ministry of Health and Long-Term Care

- Marsha Barnes, Chair of the National CDM Conference Steering Committee of the Ontario Ministry of Health and Long-Term Care, for leadership and guidance

- The National CDM Conference Planning and Coordination Team
  - Vena Persaud, Senior Manager (Acting), Primary Health Care Program Design & Development, Ontario Ministry of Health and Long-Term Care
  - Kavita Mehta, Senior Program Consultant (Acting), Primary Health Care Program Design & Development, Ontario Ministry of Health and Long-Term Care
  - Francesca Grosso, Consultant, Grosso Group, CDM Conference Project Lead

- The Chair of the National CDM Conference, Michael Decter, Founding Former Chair, Health Council of Canada

- The Breakout Session Moderators
  - Dr. David McCutcheon, CEO, Gibraltar Health Authority
  - Dr. Jim MacLean, Lead, Primary Health Care Reform, Ontario Ministry of Health and Long-Term Care
  - Dr. David Gass, Senior Advisor, Continuing and Primary Health Care, Health Canada
  - Dr. Chris Rauscher, Chair, Province-wide Chronic Disease Collaborative for Patients with Congestive Heart Failure in British Columbia
  - Louise Rosborough, Manager (Acting), Primary and Continuing Health Care Division, Health Canada

- The Breakout Session Notetakers
  - Dr. Harvey Blankenstein, Medical Consultant, Ontario Ministry of Health and Long-Term Care
  - Diane Hindman, Pharmacist Consultant, Ontario Ministry of Health and Long-Term Care
  - Barbara Roston, Manager (Acting), Primary Health Care Design and Projects, Ontario Ministry of Health and Long-Term Care
  - Vena Persaud, Senior Manager (Acting), Primary Health Care Program Design & Development, Ontario Ministry of Health and Long-Term Care

- The Canadian Federal/Provincial/Territorial Advisory Group for their support and facilitation of Canada-wide project nominations and key stakeholder participation in the conference
  - Nancy Swainson, Director (Acting), Primary Health Care Division, Health Canada
  - Cindy Moriarty, Manager, Primary Health Care Transition Fund, Health Canada
  - Valerie Tregillus, Executive Director, Chronic Disease Management and Primary Health Care Renewal, British Columbia Ministry of Health Services
  - Marnie Bell, Primary Community Services Manager, Greater Northwest Territories Health and Social Services

- · Jan Horton, Policy Analyst, Yukon Health and Social Services, Government of Yukon
- · Gogi Greeley, Primary Health Care Implementation Coordinator, Nunavut Department of Health and Social Services
- · Betty Jeffers, Senior Manager, Primary Health Care Unit, Alberta Health and Wellness
- · Marie O'Neill, Director, Primary Health Care, Manitoba Health
- · Rick Kilarski, Consultant, Saskatchewan Primary Health Services Branch
- · Valérie Fontaine, Direction des affaires intergouvernementales et de la coopération internationale, Ministère de la Santé et des Services sociaux
- · Lise Girard, Advisor, Health Care Renewal, Health & Wellness, Government of New Brunswick
- · Paula M. English, Manager, Primary Health Care, Nova Scotia Department of Health
- · Donna MacAusland, Coordinator, Primary Health Care Redesign, Prince Edward Island Department of Health and Social Services
- · Juanita Barrett, Team Leader, Office of Primary Health Care, Newfoundland and Labrador Department of Health and Community Services

• All the international keynote plenary speakers and the Breakout Session presenters from across Canada, and the many people who participated directly in the conference as organizers and enthusiastic participants

GLOSSARY OF MEDICAL TERMS

A1C (HbA1C): A1C is the newest abbreviation for HbA1C, which refers to the "glycosylated haemoglobin" molecule. A1C is a test that measures the amount of sugar that "sticks" to red blood cells. As red blood cells live for an average of 3 months, this test provides a reliable measure of the average blood sugar over a 3-month period. A1C is the best single blood test for predicting long-term adverse outcomes.

ACE inhibitor: ACE (angiotensin-converting enzyme) inhibitors are pharmacological agents that lower blood pressure by blocking angiotensin II, a potent chemical that causes blood vessels to contract. ACE inhibitors are used for the prevention of nephropathy (kidney disease) in diabetes as well as for high blood pressure and congestive heart failure.

Antiplatelets: Antiplatelet drugs are a group of powerful medications used in heart disease treatment that prevent the formation of blood clots.

ARB: Angiotensin receptor blockers (ARBs) are also medications that block the action of angiotensin II, so that blood vessels dilate and the blood pressure is reduced.

ASA: Commonly called aspirin, ASA (acetylsalicylic acid) is a common pain reliever. It is also used in small doses to prevent heart attacks or strokes.

B-blocker: Beta blockers are a class of drugs that inhibit the "sympathetic" portion of the autonomic (involuntary) nervous system. Beta blockers are commonly used to treat abnormal heart rhythms (cardiac arrhythmias) and loss of vision in glaucoma.

Creatinine: Creatinine is a by-product of metabolism that acts as an estimation of kidney function. Excess serum creatinine is an indication of advanced kidney diseases.

Dyslipidemia: Dyslipidemia is a disorder of lipoprotein metabolism, involving either excess or deficient concentration in the blood. Dyslipidemia may be manifested as elevation of total cholesterol, elevation of "bad" (LDL) cholesterol, elevation of triglyceride concentration, or decrease in "good" (HDL) cholesterol.

Echocardiography: A noninvasive diagnostic test to show the functioning of the cardiac muscle.

GHQ: The General Health Questionnaire (GHQ) screens for non-psychotic psychiatric disorders and is available in 60-, 30-, 28- and 12-item versions.

Glucometer: A glucometer is a battery-operated device used primarily by diabetic patients for testing blood glucose.

HDL: High-density lipoprotein (HDL) is commonly called "good cholesterol." It is a small circulating fat-protein molecule that carries cholesterol from the body's tissues to the liver to be metabolized and eliminated.

LDL: Low-density lipoprotein (LDL), commonly called "bad cholesterol," is a large fat-protein molecule that carries cholesterol in the cardiovascular system, occasionally adhering to the walls of vessels and causing circulatory problems.

Lipids: Lipids are organic compounds essential for the structure and function of living cells. The two main lipids in the blood are cholesterol and triglyceride.

Microalbumin screening: This diagnostic test for detecting even very low urinary albumin (protein) levels is used as a screening test for kidney disease (nephropathy) in diabetic patients.

Myocardial infarction: Commonly known as a heart attack, myocardial infarction is a disease state that occurs when the blood supply to a part of the heart is interrupted, causing damage and potential death of heart tissue.

Nephropathy: Damage to or disease of the kidney; also called nephrosis.

Neuropathy: Any disease that affects the nervous system. In common usage, it is short for *peripheral neuropathy,* meaning a disease of the peripheral nervous system.

PHQ-9: A 9-item depression scale of the Patient Health Questionnaire, PHQ-9 assists primary care clinicians in diagnosing depression as well as selecting and monitoring treatment.

Pre- and post-prandial glucometer values: Glucometer reading before and after a meal.

Retinopathy: A general term that refers to non-inflammatory damage to the retina of the eye. Most commonly it is a problem with the blood supply that causes this condition.

SF-8: The SF-8™ Health Survey is a brief, comprehensive population health survey. It has 8 items designed to track general health and ability to conduct usual activities.

Spirometry: Spirometry, literally the measurement of breath, is the most common pulmonary function test, measuring the volume and/or speed of air that can be inhaled and exhaled. Spirometry is an important tool used for assessing conditions such as asthma, pulmonary fibrosis, and COPD (chronic obstructive pulmonary disease).

Statins: Statins are pharmacological agents used in the management of disorders of lipid imbalance. They can be used alone or in conjunction with dietary therapy for primary or secondary prevention of cardiovascular disease.

Total cholesterol (TC): Total cholesterol is the total amount of all forms of cholesterol—both high-density (HDL) "good" cholesterol and low-density (LDL) "bad" cholesterol. It is used together with the HDL level to calculate the TC/HDL ratio, a key target when working toward the primary or secondary prevention of heart disease.

BIOGRAPHIES

ELIZABETH BADLEY is an epidemiologist and a health services researcher. She is a Professor in the Department of Public Health Sciences at the University of Toronto, and a Senior Scientist and Head of the Division of Outcomes and Population Health at the Toronto Western Hospital Research Institute. Dr. Badley has published widely on the epidemiology of rheumatic disorders, their impact in the population, and implications for service provision. She is the Director of the Arthritis Community Research and Evaluation Unit, Toronto, and is providing the lead in the evaluation of the Getting a Grip on Arthritis project.

JUANITA BARRETT is Team Leader, Office of Primary Health Care, Newfoundland and Labrador Department of Health and Community Services. Throughout her career, Juanita has worked in senior positions in a broad range of service areas in different jurisdictions. She is a nurse with a Master's of Business Administration, a Certified Health Executive with the Canadian College of Health Services Executives, and a surveyor with the Canadian Council on Health Services Accreditation. In all areas, Juanita has worked with restructuring, program management, regionalization, planning, change management, quality improvement, and research activities. A strong focus on client/patient service delivery is supported by an ongoing vision of facilitating quality improvement.

MARY J. BELL is Associate Professor of Medicine at the University of Toronto and Division Head and Staff Rheumatologist, Division of Rheumatology, Department of Medicine at Sunnybrook Health Sciences Centre. She has a master's degree in Design, Measurement and Evaluation from McMaster University. Dr. Bell is the Director of Continuing Education in the Department of Medicine, University of Toronto, and is also a research scientist in the Arthritis Community Research and Evaluation Unit. She is the National Director of the Patient Partners® in Arthritis Program and was scientific advisor to the Getting a Grip on Arthritis project funded by Health Canada.

ELIZABETH BODNAR is Senior Manager, Corporate Relations and Privacy, at Sault Ste. Marie's Group Health Centre (GHC). She has been at GHC for 18 years, where she is responsible for privacy, corporate and media relations, medical records, and GHC's Trust Fund. She is Past President of the Health Care Public Relations Association of Canada, and a member of the Canadian

Association of Professional Access and Privacy Administrators, International Association of Business Communicators, Canadian Health Information Management Association, Northeastern Ontario Telehealth Advisory Committee, and the Canadian Patient Safety Institute's Information and Communications Advisory Committee. Locally, Elizabeth is on the joint GHC/Sault Area Hospital Research Ethics Board, the hospital's Advance Directives Committee, and Sault Ste. Marie's Mayor's Award Committee.

JENNIFER BOYLE received her PhD degree in cartilage tissue engineering in the Department of Cellular and Molecular Pathology, Faculty of Medicine, at the University of Toronto in 1999. In her most recent position, she was a research associate with the Arthritis Community Research and Evaluation Unit in Toronto, and managed the national evaluation of the primary health care educational program, Getting a Grip on Arthritis. Dr. Boyle's research interests include client-centred care, arthritis and employment, psychosocial aspects of chronic disease, and primary health-care provider education.

BRENDAN CARR, MD, is an academic emergency physician and holds the position of Director, Primary Care, Capital District Health Authority, in Halifax, NS. Here, he is charged with leading the development and implementation of Capital Health's primary health care renewal strategy. Dr. Carr leads a team that has planned and implemented over 20 initiatives and programs over the past 4 years. Dr. Carr has a Bachelor of Science, Doctor of Medicine, and Master of Business Administration, all from Dalhousie University, Halifax. He is also working towards his Certified Health Executive designation from the Canadian College of Health Services Executives.

BEN CHAN is the inaugural Chief Executive Officer of the Health Quality Council (HQC) in Saskatchewan. The HQC has a unique mandate to both report publicly on quality of care and support quality improvement activities, and has deployed successful projects in reducing wait times, improving drug management, and reducing harm to patients. In 2006, the HQC received the Saskatchewan Health Excellence Award for its pioneering work, and Dr. Chan was named Canada's Outstanding Young Health Executive by the Canadian College of Health Service Executives, and Distinguished Alumnus of the Year by Victoria College, University of Toronto.

Dr. Chan is a former senior scientist with the Institute for Clinical Evaluative Sciences in Toronto, and has authored over 50 publications on human resource planning in health care, physician practice patterns, and primary care. He has worked as a locum family doctor and emergency department physician in over 60 rural communities and 8 provinces and territories across Canada. He holds a Bachelor of Science and MD (Toronto), Master of Public Health (Harvard), and Master of Public Affairs (Princeton).

ANN COLBOURNE, an Associate Professor of Medicine at Memorial University in St. John's, NL, and provincial physician specialist lead for Chronic

Disease Prevention and Management, has an active clinical practice in chronic disease prevention and management including a large practice in diabetes care. She has educational roles in support of primary health care teams as well as medicine, pharmacy, and nurse practitioner programs. Dr. Colbourne, a Rhodes Scholar, is a recipient of the 2006 Canadian Association for Medical Education Certificate of Merit Award. Through advocacy for and active involvement in corporate and provincial initiatives in health systems restructuring, Dr. Colbourne imparts her passion and vision for opportunities for education and service delivery for healthier individuals in healthier communities.

JAFNA COX, MD, is the Director of Research in the Division of Cardiology, Dalhousie University. His research interests relate to cardiovascular health services, outcomes, and disease management and, more recently, to cardiovascular disease prevention. He was a consultant to the Government of New Brunswick regarding provincial tertiary cardiac services, and currently serves as the Scientific Advisor to the Government of Nova Scotia's cardiovascular care program, Cardiovascular Health Nova Scotia. As a past Chair of the Scientific Program Committee of the Canadian Cardiovascular Society, Dr. Cox was responsible for organizing the largest annual scientific meeting of cardiovascular health care providers in Canada.

DAVID CROOKSTON is a family physician in Sault Ste. Marie, ON, and is on active staff at the Sault Area Hospital. He is a Fellow of the College of Family Physicians of Canada. At the Group Health Centre in Sault Ste. Marie, he is a board member of the Algoma District Medical Group, lead physician and chair of the Health Promotion Initiatives Team, and principal investigator of the Vascular Intervention Project. As Assistant Professor in the Department of Family and Community Medicine at the University of Toronto, Dr. Crookston teaches residents and medical students in his practice and chairs a planning committee of the new Northern Ontario Medical School. Other professional roles include medical professional development coordinator of the Northeastern Ontario Medical Education Corporation and chair of its Faculty Development Committee, as well as local medical director of the Northern Ontario Telehealth Network and chair of its Northeastern Ontario Steering Committee.

SANDRA DELON is the Director of Chronic Disease Management in the Calgary Health Region. She is responsible for developing a regional strategic and implementation plan for chronic disease management across the continuum of care. Sandra has worked with the Calgary Health Region for almost 10 years in a research and evaluation capacity. In addition to health care, Sandra has worked in strategic planning in a variety of sectors including management consulting with KPMG in Australia, financial services with American Express in New York, and marketing with J. Walter Thompson Advertising Agency in New York. She has been an adjunct professor at the University of South Australia, and at New York University, and currently holds this role with the University of Calgary in the Faculty of Medicine. Sandra obtained a Master of Psychology in Adelaide, Australia, and a PhD at the University of Alberta, Edmonton.

JOHN DORLAND is a health economist who recently retired as Assistant Professor in the Department of Community Health and Epidemiology, and in the School of Policy Studies at Queen's University. He was a founding member of the Queen's Centre for Health Services and Policy Research. His primary interests are the cost-effectiveness of health services, economic incentives inherent in health systems' funding and, latterly, program evaluation of primary health care reforms.

ANGELA ESTEY is the Planning Director with the Office of Regional Health Services Planning and Information, Capital Health, in Edmonton, Alberta. She also has an appointment as Associate Professor with the Faculty of Nursing, University of Alberta. With over 15 years of experience in health care, Angela has worked in a variety of positions including administration and service delivery planning within different sectors of the health care system. Much of her work has focused on integration and change management in both the acute and primary care sectors. Angela has held various leadership positions, including business lead for the design and implementation of a chronic disease information management system. Currently, she has planning lead for a regional chronic disease management integration initiative. Angela serves on many regional and provincial committees related to chronic disease management.

NADINE HENNINGSEN is the Executive Director of the Canadian Home Care Association, and is involved in national projects that support advocacy, awareness, and enhancement of home care across Canada. Nadine is active on many home care initiatives and has given presentations to federal commissions, senate committees, and provincial planning groups on home care related topics. Nadine graduated from the University of Ottawa in 1984 where she received a baccalaureate degree in science with a specialty in molecular genetics. In 2003, Nadine was awarded the Queens' Jubilee Medal for outstanding contribution to home care across Canada.

MICHAEL HINDMARSH is the President of Hindsight Healthcare Strategies, a health-care improvement consulting firm, and former Associate Director of Clinical Improvement at the MacColl Institute for Healthcare Innovation at Group Health Cooperative of Puget Sound, Washington. During his 15 years with Group Health, Mike managed federally funded research studies and directed various internal clinical improvement efforts including the creation of one of the first electronic registries for chronic disease in the United States. Along with Ed Wagner, MD, Mike and his colleagues created the Chronic Care Model, a system redesign strategy to improve the care of chronically ill patients. His current work involves design and development of a dissemination strategy for implementing the Chronic Care Model in the United States, Canada, and the United Kingdom.

NICK KATES is Professor and Vice Chair of the Department of Psychiatry and Behavioural Neurosciences at McMaster University with a cross-appointment in the Department of Family Medicine. He is also program director of the Hamilton Family Health Team. For 12 years he was the director of the Hamilton HSO Mental Health and Nutrition Program. Dr. Kates is the provincial lead for the Quality Management Collaborative, which assists Family Health Teams in Ontario to build teams and develop programs.

RICHARD LEWANCZUK is the Regional Medical Director for Chronic Disease Management for the Capital Health Region encompassing Edmonton and area. In this portfolio he oversees regional service delivery in cardiovascular risk, heart failure, diabetes, obesity, and other areas. He is a professor in both the Departments of Medicine (Division of Endocrinology) and Physiology at the University of Alberta. Dr. Lewanczuk obtained his MD from the University of Alberta in 1983 and his specialty certification in internal medicine in 1988. This was followed by a combined PhD/Endocrine Fellowship, which was completed in 1992. Dr. Lewanczuk is the immediate Past President of the Canadian Hypertension Society.

SYDNEY LINEKER is a physiotherapist with a master's degree in Design, Measurement and Evaluation from McMaster University, Hamilton. She is a research investigator with the Arthritis Community Research and Evaluation Unit, an Associate Professor in the School of Rehabilitation Science at McMaster University, and a lecturer in the School of Physical Therapy at the University of Toronto. Sydney's research interests are in the areas of health professional education, behaviour change, and knowledge transfer. She is Director of Research with the Arthritis Society, Ontario Division, and was director of the Getting a Grip on Arthritis project funded by Health Canada.

ART MACGREGOR, MD, graduated from the University of British Columbia in 1958 and has practised in Victoria since 1961. Since the early 1960s he has been interested in medical education, and served as director of intern training from 1965 to 1988. Following that he devoted himself to continuing medical education. This led to an interest in quality improvement in the early 1990s, when he fell under the spell of Donald Berwick and later Dr. Edward Wagner, the father of the Chronic Care Model.

From 1991 to 1999 Dr. Macgregor was the Chief of the Department of Family Practice in Victoria, and this opportunity allowed him to organize a group of family practitioners to take part in the first Institute for Healthcare Improvement chronic diseases collaborative in 1998. This is turn led to the 2003 Vancouver Island Health Authority (VIHA) Health Transition Fund CDM Collaborative, which has been attempting to improve the care of people with diabetes, congestive heart failure, and depression.

The VIHA collaborative was the 2003 Quality Award winner of the Canadian College of Health Executives. Dr. Macgregor was also the Canadian Diabetes Association winner of the 2005 Charles H. Best Award for outstanding contributions to the care of people with diabetes in Canada.

Along the way Dr. Macgregor was president of the national College of Family Physicians and, in 2003, was named BC's Family Physician of the Year. He is currently the consultant in chronic disease management for VIHA, and the government representative on the General Practitioners' Services Committee, which is responsible for determining incentive fees, and so on, for family physicians in BC.

MARG MCALISTER was the Canadian Home Care Association's Project Manager for the National Home Care and Primary Health Care Partnership Project, a 2½-year initiative that demonstrated the value of home care within primary health care renewal through participants from Calgary, Alberta, and Halton/Peel, Ontario. She is a registered nurse and graduate of the Canadian Institute of Management. Marg's experience spans the acute and home care sectors where she has held a variety of positions including staff nurse, middle manager, and senior executive. Marg also provides consulting services to the home care industry and has supported the authoring of a number of related papers and reports.

MARY ANN MCCOLL is the Associate Director, Research, at the Centre for Health Services and Policy Research, and a Professor in the Department of Community Health and Epidemiology and in the School of Rehabilitation Therapy at Queen's University. She received a PhD in Preventive Medicine and Biostatistics from the University of Toronto in 1991, and a Master's in Community Health and Epidemiology in 1983. From 1987 to 1992, she was Director of Research at Lyndhurst Spinal Cord Centre. Her primary research interests are health services and policy for people with disabilities, community integration and social support for people with disabilities, and measurement issues in disability and rehabilitation. She has been involved in a number of projects on access to primary care for people with disabilities. Dr. McColl is a member of the Ontario Ministry of Health and Long-Term Care's Family Health Team Advisory Group, and the Chronic Disease Management Task Force.

PATRICK MCGOWAN is an Associate Professor with the University of Victoria – Centre on Aging. His doctorate degree is in health promotion research. His research career over the last 25 years has focused on aspects of health education programs for chronic health conditions. He has been implementing and researching self-management programs relating to particular chronic health conditions such as diabetes, arthritis, osteoarthritis, and tuberculosis. As well, he has been researching the feasibility, viability, acceptability, and effectiveness of a general self-management program called the Chronic Disease Self-Management Program, which is offered to persons experiencing any type of chronic health condition. This research is being conducted at the community, provincial, national, and international levels. Dr. McGowan is based in Delta, BC, where he directs the University of Victoria, Centre on Aging – Ladner Satellite Office.

MIKKI MILLAR graduated from Montana State University–Northern with an Associates Degree of Science in Nursing. She has been practising as an RN for 11 years, with 3 years in emergency and ICU and the remaining time in rural nursing. Mikki has equal experience working on both sides of the U.S./ Canada border, giving her a working knowledge of both types of health care delivery. She worked extensively in Montana with mid-level practitioners in an acute setting, where she was introduced to primary health care. Mikki completed her Primary Care Nurse Practitioner certificate in May 2004 through the Saskatchewan Institute of Applied Science and Technology, and began her employment in that role with the Cypress Health Region in January 2005. She works primarily out of the Leader Medical Clinic, with a satellite clinic in Eatonia one day a week. Her work at present is half clinical and half community-focused, with an emphasis on prevention and health promotion.

PAUL NYHOF is Director of the Provincial Health Contact Centre, operator of Health Links – Info Sante. He has held call centre management positions at Reach Canada (a division of CanWest Global) and Manitoba Public Insurance. He served as part of the National Call Centre team at Stentor Resource Centre and has served in an executive capacity on the board of the Manitoba Call Centre Association. He is a doctoral candidate in Business Administration (Management), holds a Master of Science in Administration (Human Resources) from Central Michigan University, and a Bachelor of Arts from the University of Winnipeg (Political Science/Justice & Law Enforcement). He teaches in the Faculty of Management at the I.H. Asper School of Business at the University of Manitoba.

BLAIR O'NEILL, MD, is Professor and Head, Division of Cardiology, Dalhousie University and Chief of Service, Queen Elizabeth II Health Sciences Centre, Halifax. His research interests have been related to primary and secondary prevention, endothelial dysfunction and its treatment, reduction of restenosis following percutaneous interventions, and improvement in technologies related to interventional cardiology. Dr. O'Neill is interested in improving access to cardiovascular procedures, and closing care gaps along the continuum of patient care. He has been Chair of the Medical Devices Committee of the Canadian Cardiovascular Society for the past 5 years, and was recently appointed Chair of the Access to Care Committee of the Canadian Cardiovascular Society.

REBECCA ROSEN works half-time as a Fellow in Health Policy at the King's Fund and half-time as a GP in South East London. Her work on the management of people with long-term conditions spans national policy analysis and the development of better local services. Current projects include work with selected London primary care trusts on developing services to reduce hospital admissions, international comparisons of models of care for people with complex chronic health and social care needs, and qualitative studies of patient and GP views on choice in health care. Dr. Rosen's other interests include the development of new professional roles in primary care, the impact of GPs with special clinical interests on access to care, and the future of medical professionalism. She is also a trustee of Asthma UK, and chair of a small charity promoting dialogue and understanding between artists and scientists.

JOSHUA SEIDMAN leads the independent, not-for-profit Center for Information Therapy (Ix Center) in Bethesda, MD, applying his extensive experience in strategic planning, product development, research, and education. Before joining the IxCenter, he served as senior editor and director of quality initiatives for the Advisory Board Company's consumer health initiative. Dr. Seidman has also worked for the National Committee for Quality Assurance as the director of measure development, and as assistant director of private sector relations at the American College of Cardiology, where he conducted extensive research and analysis in managed care, quality-of-care issues, and other aspects of the health care industry. Dr. Seidman holds a PhD in health services research and a Master's of Health Science in health policy and management, both from the Johns Hopkins School of Public Health.

MARIANNE STEWART is Vice President and Chief Operating Officer for Capital Health's Primary Care Division. She holds a Bachelor of Nursing Science degree, Queen's University, and a Master's in Health Sciences Administration, University of Alberta. Marianne has strategic and operational lead for the division, establishing evidence-based primary care services that are continually adjusted to meet changing population needs. Marianne also has the lead for implementing primary health care reform—including the new trilateral agreement with Alberta Medical Association and Alberta Health and Wellness—and implementing chronic disease management for the Capital Health Region, Alberta.

CLAUDINE SZPILFOGEL, ANCHOR Project Manager, has extensive experience in the pharmaceutical and health sectors. She has worked as a research and health consultant in both the public and private sectors. Her experience includes public-private partnerships, large-scale project management, research design, instrument development and evaluation, and applying research to planning. Claudine is also experienced in managing the transition of primary care practices to comprehensive primary health care models, including the development of practice plans, deliverables, and governance structures. Claudine has a Bachelor of Science in Kinesiology and a Master's in Community Health and Epidemiology, both from Dalhousie University, Halifax, NS. She is a partner of Research Power Inc.

SHANNON TURNER is Manager, Health Promotion and Clinical Prevention, for the Vancouver Island Health Authority. Under the Primary Health Care Transition Fund, Shannon served as provincial coordinator for the BC Primary Health Prevention Support Program. Shannon has worked across the health care continuum for over 20 years, providing decision support, health promotion, program management, information management, risk management, quality improvement, and strategic planning services. She holds a Bachelor of Arts in History, a Bachelor of Science in Health Informatics, and a Master of Science in Public Health—International Health. Shannon has experience at all levels of governance from local through to international program support. Shannon is currently President of the Public Health Association of BC and is committed to health system reform.

MICHAEL VALLIS, PhD, is a Registered Clinical Health Psychologist at the Queen Elizabeth II Health Sciences Centre, and Associate Professor, Dalhousie University, Halifax. He qualified in 1983 and has worked in Toronto (1983–88) and Halifax (1988–present). His area of expertise is in adult health psychology, with an emphasis on diabetes, gastroenterology, cardiovascular risk, and obesity. Dr. Vallis maintains an active clinical practice as well as a research program and teaches regularly within the hospital and university. He is active at a national level within organizations such as the Canadian Diabetes Association and Obesity Canada, and regularly serves as a consultant to industry on behaviour change.

PAUL WALLACE, MD, is an active participant, program leader, and perpetual student in clinical quality improvement, especially in the areas of performance measurement, evidence-based medicine, and disease management. As Medical Director of Health and Productivity Management Programs in Kaiser Permanente's (KP) national Permanente federation based in Oakland, CA, he leads work to extend KP's experience with population-based care to further develop and integrate wellness, health maintenance, and productivity enhancement interventions. He was the Executive Director of Kaiser Permanente's Care Management Institute (CMI) from 2000 to 2005, and continues as a Senior Advisor to CMI and to KP Healthy Solutions, the KP disease management company established in 2005. Dr. Wallace, an internist and hematologist, joined Kaiser Permanente in 1989, and has participated in its program-wide new technology, research, guidelines, and diversity committees. He is a member of the American National Advisory Council for the Agency of Healthcare Research and Quality, the Institute of Medicine Board on Population Health and Public Health Practice, the Medical Coverage Advisory Committee for the Center for Medicare and Medicaid Services, and the Committee on Performance Measurement for the National Committee for Quality Assurance. He is the Board Chair of the Center for Information Therapy, and is also a board member of the Disease Management Association of America (DMAA). In 2004 he was recognized by the DMAA with the Karen Coughlin Individual Disease Management Leadership Award.

Queen's Policy Studies
Recent Publications

The Queen's Policy Studies Series is dedicated to the exploration of major public policy issues that confront governments and society in Canada and other nations.

Our books are available from good bookstores everywhere, including the Queen's University bookstore (http://www.campusbookstore.com/). McGill-Queen's University Press is the exclusive world representative and distributor of books in the series. A full catalogue and ordering information may be found on their web site (http://mqup.mcgill.ca/).

School of Policy Studies

Fulfilling Potential, Creating Success: Perspectives on Human Capital Development,
Garnett Picot, Ron Saunders and Arthur Sweetman (eds.), 2007
Paper ISBN 1-55339-127-6   Cloth ISBN 1-55339-128-4

Reinventing Canadian Defence Procurement: A View from the Inside, Alan S. Williams, 2006
Paper ISBN 0-9781693-0-1 (Published in association with Breakout Educational Network)

SARS in Context: Memory, History, Policy, Jacalyn Duffin and Arthur Sweetman (eds.), 2006
Paper ISBN 0-7735-3194-7 Cloth ISBN 0-7735-3193-9 (Published in association with McGill-Queen's University Press)

Dreamland: How Canada's Pretend Foreign Policy has Undermined Sovereignty, Roy Rempel, 2006
Paper ISBN 1-55339-118-7 Cloth ISBN 1-55339-119-5 (Published in association with Breakout Educational Network)

Canadian and Mexican Security in the New North America: Challenges and Prospects,
Jordi Díez (ed.), 2006   Paper ISBN 1-55339-123-3 Cloth ISBN 1-55339-122-7

Global Networks and Local Linkages: The Paradox of Cluster Development in an Open Economy, David A. Wolfe and Matthew Lucas (eds.), 2005
Paper ISBN 1-55339-047-4 Cloth ISBN 1-55339-048-2

Choice of Force: Special Operations for Canada, David Last and Bernd Horn (eds.), 2005
Paper ISBN 1-55339-044-X Cloth ISBN 1-55339-045-8

Force of Choice: Perspectives on Special Operations, Bernd Horn, J. Paul de B. Taillon, and David Last (eds.), 2004   Paper ISBN 1-55339-042-3 Cloth 1-55339-043-1

New Missions, Old Problems, Douglas L. Bland, David Last, Franklin Pinch, and Alan Okros (eds.), 2004   Paper ISBN 1-55339-034-2 Cloth 1-55339-035-0

The North American Democratic Peace: Absence of War and Security Institution-Building in Canada-US Relations, 1867-1958, Stéphane Roussel, 2004
Paper ISBN 0-88911-937-6 Cloth 0-88911-932-2

Implementing Primary Care Reform: Barriers and Facilitators, Ruth Wilson, S.E.D. Shortt and John Dorland (eds.), 2004   Paper ISBN 1-55339-040-7 Cloth 1-55339-041-5

Social and Cultural Change, David Last, Franklin Pinch, Douglas L. Bland, and Alan Okros (eds.), 2004   Paper ISBN 1-55339-032-6 Cloth 1-55339-033-4

Clusters in a Cold Climate: Innovation Dynamics in a Diverse Economy, David A. Wolfe and Matthew Lucas (eds.), 2004   Paper ISBN 1-55339-038-5 Cloth 1-55339-039-3